Musculoskeletal
Imaging

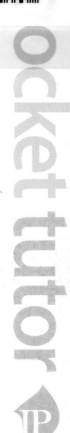

Pocket tutor

D1354061

Musculoskeletal Imaging

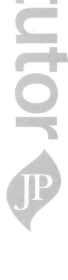

Teik Chooi Oh MBBCh BAO AFRCSI FRCR
Consultant Musculoskeletal and Radionuclide
Radiologist
Honorary Lecturer
Lancashire Teaching Hospitals NHS Trust
Preston, UK

Matthew Budak MD FRCR
Specialty Registrar in Clinical Radiology
Ninewells Hospital and Medical School
Dundee, UK

Rakesh Mehan MBChB FRCR
Consultant Radiologist
Bolton Hospital NHS Foundation Trust
Bolton, UK

JP
medical
publishers

© 2014 JP Medical Ltd.

Published by JP Medical Ltd, 83 Victoria Street, London, SW1H 0HW, UK

Tel: +44 (0)20 3170 8910   Fax: +44 (0)20 3008 6180

Email: info@jpmedpub.com   Web: www.jpmedpub.com

ISBN: 978-1-907816-68-0

British Library Cataloguing in Publication Data
A catalogue record for this book is available from the British Library

Library of Congress Cataloging in Publication Data
A catalog record for this book is available from the Library of Congress

JP Medical Ltd is a subsidiary of Jaypee Brothers Medical Publishers (P) Ltd, New Delhi, India

Publisher:	Richard Furn
Development Editors:	Paul Mayhew, Thomas Fletcher
Design:	Designers Collective Ltd

Typeset, printed and bound in India.

Foreword

Knowledge of musculoskeletal disorders and their typical radiological appearances is relevant to many clinicians and all radiologists – not just those with a special interest in musculoskeletal imaging – throughout their training and career.

Pocket Tutor Musculoskeletal Imaging begins by covering the technical principles of the different imaging methods applied to the skeleton, includinsg radiographs, ultrasound, computed tomography, magnetic resonance imaging and radionuclide scans. It then describes what is seen in normal and abnormal musculoskeletal tissues using each modality. Next, taking an anatomical approach and including a wealth of annotated images, the authors provide concise descriptions of the most common disorders of each region, the optimum imaging technique and the standard treatment. There is significant coverage of trauma in each regional chapter, making the book particularly relevant to those working in emergency and orthopaedic departments. The final chapter describes the radiological patterns seen with bone tumours and infarcts, osteomyelitis, rickets, arthritis, and osteochondritis dissicans.

Readers are offered a sound basis on which to diagnose the common and classical disorders affecting the skeleton, including knowledge of the optimum imaging method for identification. The authors have described and illustrated musculoskeletal pathology in an admirably succinct and informative way.

Professor Judith Adams
Consultant Radiologist, Manchester Royal Infirmary
Honorary Professor of Diagnostic Radiology
University of Manchester
Manchester, UK

Preface

Imaging of the musculoskeletal system often intimidates students and trainees, and it can even be daunting for more experienced clinicians. A thorough grasp of radiological anatomy and an appreciation of underlying principles will help overcome this and provide a foundation for interpreting the imaging results seen in practice. *Pocket Tutor Musculoskeletal Imaging* has been written to help you develop this knowledge and understanding.

The book opens by demonstrating the appearance of normal tissues before going on to illustrate the radiological features of pathological tissues. Having provided a framework for recognising normal findings and key abnormal signs, subsequent chapters summarise the radiological anatomy, clinical appearance and management of the most common musculoskeletal diseases, by body region. A final chapter demonstrates common systemic pathologies which are not easily grouped into a single region. All chapters are lavishly illustrated with high-quality, clearly labelled images.

We hope that this book helps you develop the skills required to interpret images of musculoskeletal presentations.

Teik Chooi Oh
Matthew Budak
Rakesh Mehan
February 2014

Contents

Acknowledgements

I wish to thank my colleagues at the Royal Preston & Chorley Hospital and the South Ribble Hospital for their encouragement and for providing a fantastic working environment. I am especially grateful to Dr Priam Heire for his invaluable aid in the anatomy sections.

I extend my gratitude to all the staff at JP Medical, in particular Paul Mayhew, for his patience and guidance throughout the process.

TCO

I would like to thank Dr Barry Oliver, Dr Naveena Thomas and Dr Christine Walker for their MSK mentorship during my specialist training at Ninewells Hospital and Medical School. Their hard work, patience and dedication for teaching will always be remembered.

MB

I wish to thank Dr Jeremy Jenkins and Dr Richard Whitehouse for their invaluable advice and support.

RM

Dedication

This book is dedicated to my parents, Oh Khay Seng and Gan Poh Kooi, who have always supported me in my lifelong ambition to be a doctor.

TCO

For Tilly and Karo.

MB

Understanding normal results

Only by understanding normal findings can you develop the skills to identify abnormal results and correctly diagnose the condition causing them. In radiology, various imaging modalities are used; each has its own way of producing an image. Knowing the basic concepts underlying the different types of radiological examination will enable you to interpret the images produced and understand the pathological processes occurring, even if the actual diagnosis is unknown.

1.1 Plain radiography

The **plain radiograph** remains an important and useful diagnostic tool. This is especially true in musculoskeletal radiology, as radiographs are quick, widely available and inexpensive. They are well tolerated by most, if not all, patients. Fractures and focal bony abnormalities are easily detected.

However, radiography exposes the patient to **ionising radiation in the form of X-rays**. Although the radiation burden of radiography and other radiological examinations is small (**Table 1.1**), the risk of developmental problems and lifetime cancer risk is increased. Therefore any examination must be clinically justified.

How it works

X-rays are passed through a part of the body and the resultant image is captured on an imaging plate (traditionally a film but nowadays a digital detector). The X-rays are either absorbed or scattered by the different layers of tissue. The degree of absorption or scattering depends on the density of the tissue. Thus differences in tissue density are visualised as differences in contrast in the overall image.

Examination	Equivalent period of natural background radiation	Estimated additional lifetime risk of cancer per examination
• Radiograph of chest, arms, legs, hands, feet or teeth	A few days	Negligible: < 1 in 1,000,000
• Radiograph of skull, head or neck	A few weeks	Minimal: 1 in 1,000,000 to 1 in 100,000
• Radiograph of hip, spine, abdomen or pelvis • CT of head	A few months to a year	Very low: 1 in 100,000 to 1 in 10,000
• Radiograph of kidneys and bladder (intravenous urogram) • CT of chest or abdomen	A few years	Low: 1 in 10,000 to 3 in 1000
CT, computerised tomography.		

Table 1.1 Risks of common radiological examinations

Radiographic densities

The four main classes of **radiographic density** are gas, fat, soft tissue and bone. Metal may also be seen on radiographs (**Figure 1.1**).

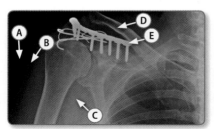

Figure 1.1 Radiograph of the right shoulder, showing five different radiographic densities in an acromial fixation: in increasing order of density, gas or air Ⓐ, fat Ⓑ, soft tissue Ⓒ, bone Ⓓ and metal Ⓔ.

Gas

Gas (not always air) has the lowest density and therefore absorbs very few X-ray photons. Most of the energy passes through areas of gas, which therefore appear black on the final image.

Fat

Fat has low density but absorbs X-ray energy slightly more than gas does. Therefore areas of fat appear a shade lighter than black, i.e. a dark grey, on the image. Dark-grey areas of fat are seen between layers of soft tissue and help delineate these layers.

Soft tissue

Soft tissue partially absorbs and scatters X-rays, resulting in a grey shadow on the image. Adjacent soft tissues of the same density are indistinguishable if there is no intervening fat, gas or metal.

Bone

Bone contains calcium, which makes it very dense. Therefore bone appears light grey to white on radiographs. The exact shade of grey depends on which part of the bone is being viewed. For example, the light grey medullary cavity is clearly distinguishable from the white cortex in a long bone.

Metal

Metal has the highest density. Its presence in the body may be intentional (e.g. when a screw fixation is used) or unintentional (e.g. in cases of a retained suture needle).

Principles of assessment of radiographs

The general principle is to use a systematic approach to assess the entire image.

- **Alignment**: check that all the bones and joints are in anatomically correct alignment. Loss of alignment can result from fractures or dislocations.
- **Bones**: check the contour of every bone by tracing around the entire cortex. Suspect a fracture if there is any step or

break in the cortex. After checking the contours, examine bone texture: the fine trabeculae of the bones should be preserved.

- **Cartilage**: cartilage is not visible on radiographs, but check that the joint spaces are present and congruent throughout the joint. Joint space narrowing or widening may indicate underlying pathology.
- **Soft tissue**: check for the presence of soft tissue changes which can indicate underlying pathology even when the bones and joints appear normal.

1.2 Ultrasound

Ultrasound is a particularly useful tool in musculoskeletal imaging, because it is good at visualising superficial structures due to the high-resolution images it generates. Also, ultrasound images of some structures, such as tendons, are more detailed than those of magnetic resonance imaging (MRI).

However, ultrasound is operator-dependent; the quality of ultrasound images and the accuracy of diagnosis is entirely dependent on the expertise of the operator, and ultrasound skills take a long time to acquire. Also, ultrasound has limited ability to visualise deeper structures or those masked by dense structures such as bone.

How it works

A pulsed wave of ultrasound (2–15 MHz) is transmitted. It loses energy as it passes through the body. The amount of energy lost depends on the amount of energy absorbed by the material. The rate of absorption depends on the type of material through which the pulse passes and the frequency of the ultrasound.

The absorption rate of a material is specified by its **attenuation coefficient**. The lower the coefficient, the more easily the ultrasound pulse penetrates the material (**Figure 1.2**). Therefore materials with a lower attenuation coefficient are more **anechoic** and look darker on ultrasound. Conversely, materials with a higher attenuation coefficient are more **echogenic** and look brighter on ultrasound.

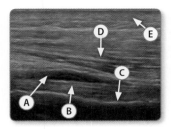

Figure 1.2 Ultrasound of the arm, showing various tissue densities: fluid Ⓐ in the tendon sheath of the long head of the biceps tendon Ⓑ, lying on the cortical bony surface Ⓒ, with overlying deltoid muscle Ⓓ and superficial subcutaneous fat Ⓔ.

Echogenicity

Fluid

Fluids are anechoic and thus appear dark on ultrasound. Different fluids, for example blood and water, have different reflective properties. Water appears totally **anechoic** or black on the screen, whereas blood pooled within a vein appears almost black on the screen, with a slight turbidity due to the cellular components within.

Fat

Fat appears as a bright (**hyperechoic**) area.

Soft tissue

Soft tissue appearances vary according to the exact type of tissue.

- **Muscle** is **hypoechoic**. In the short axis (transverse plane) it looks dark with small speckled dots (due to perimysial connective tissue within it). In the long axis (longitudinal plane) it is dark with hypoechoic cylindrical structures (fascicles), resembling parallel lines of spaghetti.
- **Tendons** have a fibrolinear pattern, seen on US as parallel lines in the longitudinal axis. In the transverse axis, tendons are round or ovoid. Tendons may be surrounded by either a synovium-lined sheath or a dense connective tissue known as the paratenon (**Figure 1.3**).
- **Ligaments** look similar to tendons. However, ligaments have a more compact fibrolinear architecture and hence more hyperechoic pattern.

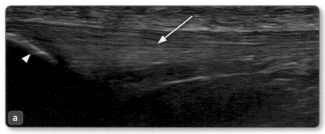

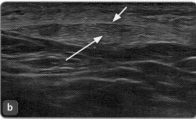

Figure 1.3 (a) Longitudinal ultrasound of the knee, showing fibrolinear parallel lines (arrow) in the patellar tendon, arising from the lower pole of the patella (arrowhead). (b) Transverse ultrasound showing the ovoid tendon (long arrow) with a thin paratenon (short arrow).

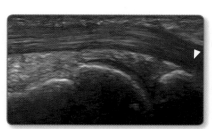

Figure 1.4 Longitudinal ultrasound of the finger, showing anisotropic artefact in the distal portion of the flexor tendon (arrowhead) as it curves away (deeper) from the probe.

Clinical insight

Be aware of **anisotropy** (**Figure 1.4**). Focal areas of hypoechogenicity appear if the ultrasound beam is not perpendicular to the structure being examined. This problem is common with curvilinear structures such as tendons. Do not mistake the hypoechoic areas for a pathological change. The artefact is removed by simply adjusting the position of the probe (**Figure 1.5**).

- **Nerves** have fascicular structures that are slightly less echogenic than tendons and ligaments.

Bone

The cortical layer of bone appears as a thin, well-defined, hyperechoic line casting an acoustic shadow deep to its surface.

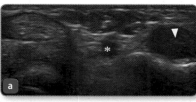

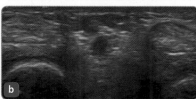

Figure 1.5 Transverse ultrasound of the fingers, showing the common flexor tendons. (a) Anisotropic artefact in the ring finger (arrowhead). A digital artery (*) lies between the tendons. (b) Anisotropy resolves (arrow) when the probe position is adjusted.

At joint surfaces, the articular cartilage appears as a thin hypoechoic rim paralleling the echogenic articular cortex.

Principles of ultrasound assessment

It is essential to use the correct ultrasound in order to produce optimal diagnostic images. Choice of probe (low or high frequency) depends on the depth of the tissue that is being reviewed. In principle, use the highest frequency probe possible for the area examined, understanding that what is gained in higher resolution is lost in reduced depth. Target the examination to a specific area, and assess all relevant structures in that area systematically and thoroughly. If an abnormality is found, use basic principles to understand which tissue is involved, and look for other changes such as vascularity and compressibility to assist in unifying the underlying diagnosis. Doppler ultrasound allows detection of vascular flow within the vessels and tissues.

1.3 Computerised tomography

Computerised tomography (CT) produces detailed cross-sectional images of the body. CT is faster to perform than MRI and has a high spatial resolution. It is used in musculoskeletal imaging primarily to assess bones and bony lesions. CT is especially useful when planning surgery for complex fractures.

Computerised tomography is well tolerated by most patients. However, it carries an even higher radiation burden than that of radiographs (**Table 1.1**). Therefore CT should be reserved for instances in which other imaging modalities cannot provide the information needed.

How it works

Computerised tomography produces images by using a series of narrow beams of X-rays, in contrast to radiography, which uses one narrow beam. A computer programme uses the obtained X-ray absorption data to generate images called **tomograms**. Each tomogram represents a cross-sectional slice of a three-dimensional structure. Modern CT uses voxels (3D pixels) to allow multi-planar reconstruction (MPR) review. Contrast material may be injected to enhance the appearance of the tissues.

Computerised tomography provides good cross-sectional images, which can be reconstructed in multiple planes. The intensity scale used in CT is related to the density of the material and is known as the **Hounsfield unit** (HU) scale.

Computerised tomography densities

As with radiographs, the key to interpreting CT scans is an understanding of the normal appearance of tissues, each demonstrating its own attenuation value. The attenuation scale ranges from -1000 HU for air or gas, through 0 HU for water and to 3000 HU for dense bone (**Figure 1.6**).

Gas

Gases, such as those in air, do not absorb X-rays emitted by the CT scanner and therefore appear black on the image.

Fat

Fat on average measures –50 HU, so on CT it appears darker than water but lighter than gas.

Fluid

Attenuation of water is 0 HU, but most fluid in the body measures approximately 15–25 HU. Fluids such as water are lighter than fat on CT.

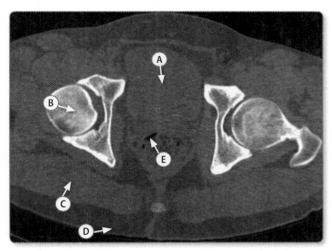

Figure 1.6 Computerised tomography of the pelvis, showing various degrees of tissue attenuation. Ⓐ Fluid in the bladder, Ⓑ bones of the pelvis and femur, Ⓒ muscles, Ⓓ subcutaneous fat. Small pockets of intraluminal gas (arrowhead) are present in the rectum.

Soft tissue

Soft tissue has a wide range of attenuation values, ranging from 30 HU for muscle to 90 HU for tendon.

Bone

Different types of bone have different attenuation values, ranging from 700 HU for cancellous bone to > 1000 HU for dense bone. Bones appear white on the normal soft tissue window setting (since all structures hyperdense to 75 HU appear white) and are best visualised on the bone window setting (centred at 300 HU, with width of 1500 HU).

Principles of CT assessment

Use a systematic approach to assess every structure separately and how each structure affects surrounding tissues. To help clinicians, describe bony fragments and their relation to each other, and provide an overall grading of the injury or disease.

1.4 Magnetic resonance imaging

Magnetic resonance imaging provides excellent contrast resolution of tissues. Therefore it is a very sensitive modality for detecting subtle or early pathology, particularly oedema, a sensitive and early suggestion of underlying pathology. MRI is now the mainstay of complex musculoskeletal imaging. MRI is also good for the local staging of bony and soft tissue tumours, because of its superb ability to differentiate tissue types.

However, there are contraindications for MRI. Magnetically activated implant devices (especially pacemakers) and ferromagnetic metals (especially in the brain or eye) are contraindications for MRI. Also, patients who are prone to claustrophobia may be unable to tolerate MRI.

How it works

In MRI, a very strong magnet is used. The magnetic field aligns hydrogen protons, whilst radiofrequency (RF) pulses disrupt their alignment. The protons then realign, giving off signals, to form images. Various **pulse sequences** are used. The two commonest sequences produce **T1-weighted** and **T2-weighted** images. T1-weighted images (**Figure 1.7a**) are generally best for showing anatomical structures. T2-weighted images (**Figure 1.7b**) are typically used to show pathological conditions.

Gadolinium contrast helps to distinguish different pathologies based on the degree of enhancement. It is **hyperintense** on T1-weighted images. T1-weighted fat-saturated images are obtained before and after gadolinium injection: in these, the fat signal is 'disrupted' by a selective radiofrequency pulse, and appears dark.

Short T1 inversion recovery (STIR) is a pulse sequence similar to that used in T2 weighting. However, in STIR sequences, an inversion recovery pulse is used to nullify the signal from the

> ## Guiding principle
>
> Typically, only five substances appear hyperintense on T1-weighted images: fat, subacute blood (i.e. methaemoglobin), melanin, proteinaceous material (e.g. mucus) and paramagnetic material (gadolinium contrast and some heavy metals).

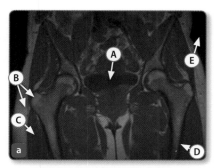

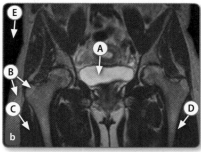

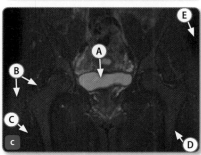

Figure 1.7 (a) T1-weighted, (b) T2-weighted and (c) short T1 inversion recovery (STIR) magnetic resonance imaging of the pelvis. Fluid in the bladder (A) is dark on the T1-weighted image but bright on the T2-weighted and STIR images. Medullary and subcutaneous fat (B) is bright on T1- and T2-weighted images but dark on the STIR image. Musculature (C) gives an intermediate signal on the T1-weighted image, appearing slightly brighter than on the T2-weighted image; it is dark on the STIR image. Cortical bone (D) and fibrous ligaments (not shown) are dark on all sequences. (E) Air or gas.

fat, so it appears **hypointense** or dark (**Figure 1.7**c). Typically, the remaining hyperintense signal is from fluid only, and this fluid signal often shows the pathological tissue. All other signal intensities remain the same. STIR is often used in musculoskeletal MRI.

Signal intensity

Because of the nature of MRI, different materials have different signals depending on the sequence used. By looking at several sequences, it is possible to identify which tissues are present (**Table 1.2**).

Gas

Gas has a low signal on all sequences because of the absence of any hydrogen atoms.

Fat

Fat is the only tissue that returns an increased signal on both T1-weighted and T2-weighted images, therefore it should always be distinguishable. STIR or fat-saturated sequences are designed to eliminate this signal, resulting in low signal from fat.

Tissue[a]	T1-weighted sequence	T2-weighted sequence
Fluid (A)	Hypointense/low (dark)	Hyperintense/high (bright)
Fat and medullary bone (B)	Hyperintense/high (bright)	Isointense/intermediate (moderate)
Muscle (C)	Isointense/intermediate (moderate)	Hypointense/low (dark)
Tendons, ligaments and fibrocartilage	Hypointense/low (dark)	Hypointense/low (dark)
Cortical bone (D)	Hypointense/low (dark)	Hypointense/low (dark)
Air or gas (E)	Hypointense/low (dark)	Hypointense/low (dark)
[a]Letters A to E correspond to labelling on Figure 1.7.		

Table 1.2 Signal intensities for various materials on T1-weighted and T2-weighted MRI sequences

Fluid

Fluid is classically hypointense on T1-weighted images and hyperintense on T2-weighted images. To help determine whether a sequence is T1 weighted or T2 weighted, always look for physiological areas of fluid, such as the bladder, the brain and spinal cord (containing cerebrospinal fluid), and the joints.

Soft tissue

The signal intensity of soft tissue on MRI depends on the amount of water it contains. Structures lacking water, such as tendons and ligaments, show no or low signal on all sequences.

Bone

Cortical bone lacks free water and so gives no signal on all sequences. However, the medullary cavity may give a fatty signal (with yellow marrow) or a more fluid signal (with red marrow).

Principles of MRI assessment

The key to assessing MRI results is to use all the various sequences and planes covering the relevant structures, and to understand the normal signal appearances of each tissue. Pathological changes can be detected by identifying the abnormal signal, which can be further distinguished in some pathologies by using gadolinium contrast.

1.5 Nuclear medicine

Nuclear medicine (radionuclide imaging) is another method of assessing certain musculoskeletal diseases. **Isotope bone scaning (bone scintigraphy)** is used specifically for detecting osteoblastic bony activity, including fractures, infection and bony tumours. More specialised tests, such as a **leucocyte-labelled study,** can be even more specific for infections, particularly those in a joint prosthesis.

Nuclear medicine is relatively expensive but widely available and very sensitive. Its high sensitivity makes it an excellent tool to exclude bony metastasis. However, it has a low spatial resolution and has low diagnostic specificity. Also, like radiography and CT, it carries a radiation burden.

How it works

The principle behind nuclear medicine is the use of a **marker** specific for the intended organ or system, attaching this marker to a radioactive **tracer**, typically a radioactive isotope. The labelled marker is injected intravenously, and travels to and is taken up by the intended organ. The isotope emits radiation when it decays: a **gamma camera** detects areas in which the tracer has localised. These so-called **hot spots** show the presence of pathological changes.

In an isotope bone scan, **methylene diphosphonate** is used as the marker because it is taken up by bone. This marker is attached to a tracer, the metastable **technetium-99m** isotope, which emits gamma rays when it decays to its stable technetium-99 form.

> ### Guiding principle
>
> Remember that unlike the other forms of imaging, nuclear medicine provides a functional test and not an anatomical one. Scans show metabolic activity in lesions but do not necessarily localise these lesions very well. Therefore it is a sensitive test but not a specific one.

Tissue visualisation
Bone

Methylene diphosphonate–technetium-99m is widely used for isotope bone scans. It is taken up throughout the skeleton, with intense uptake in the physis of the long bones due to osteoblastic activity. Marrow-containing flat facial bones in children are also hot spots.

Accumulation of the technetium-99m tracer decreases with age, but some areas shows persistent increased uptake symmetrically: the acromial and coracoid process, medial ends of the clavicle, sternomanubrial joint, sacral ala and sites of tendinous insertion (e.g. the anterior and posterior iliac spine). Areas of dental treatment also may show focal increased uptake.

The bones at the major joints, such as the shoulders and hips, show mild increased uptake symmetrically. The pattern of increased uptake at the sternoclavicular joints and manubrium sterni is variable. Further increased uptake can be present when there is arthropathy. Common degenerative (and possibly asymptomatic) arthropathic sites include the shoulders, hips, knees and smaller carpal and tarsal joints. Facet joint arthropathy may cause unilateral uptake in the spine.

A triple-phase bone scan is done for suspected infection. Normal uniform uptake is visible in all three phases if no pathological changes are present (see Chapter 2 for details). Equivocal results may indicate specialised leucocyte scanning, in which white cells harvested from the patient are labelled with a suitable isotope (usually **indium-111**) and reinjected into the patient. Accumulation of the isotope indicates local infection.

Soft tissue

Nuclear medicine is not primarily used for visualising soft tissue pathology. However, in an isotope bone scan there is physiological soft tissue uptake, and it is important not to mistake this for a pathological change. The isotope is excreted through the urinary system, so the kidneys, ureters and bladder all show increased uptake. Tracer uptake is often seen at sites of intravenous injection too. Sometimes, some unbound (free) technetium will also accumulate in the thyroid.

Principles of bone scan assessment

A good understanding of what constitutes normal uptake is needed. Look carefully for areas of increased uptake, particularly asymmetrical uptake (**Figure 1.8**). Distinguishing physiological from pathological uptake is important. It is equally important to be aware of areas of **photopaenic defect** (so-called **cold spots**). These areas often indicate loss or destruction of bone, and the pathology may lie in the cold spot. If in doubt, radiographs of the affected area can help increase the specificity of the diagnosis. Further anatomical correlation of lesions can sometimes be obtained with MRI.

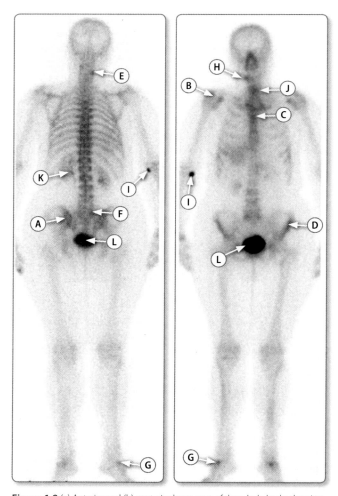

Figure 1.8 (a) Anterior and (b) posterior bone scan of the whole body, showing normal skeletal uptake, including areas of increased uptake at the sacral ala (A), coracoid (B) and sternum (C). The anterior and posterior iliac spine (D) has tendinous insertions. Focal uptake in the cervical spine (E), lumbar spine (F) and tarsal bones (G) is consistent with joint de0generation. Dental uptake is present (H). Soft tissue uptake includes that at an intravenous site (I), the thyroid (J), the renal system (K) and the bladder (L).

Recognising abnormalities

As the various imaging modalities visualise tissues differently, it is vital that the appropriate method is chosen for each patient. The suspected pathologsy determines which modality is best.

Generally, suspected bonse pathologies should first be assessed by **radiography**. For further clarification of fractures or arthropathy, **computerised tomography** (CT) is often more useful than **magnetic resonance imaging** (MRI), the latter being useful if surrounding soft tissues are involved. However, because of its high sensitivity **isotope bone scan** is the first-line investigation for widespread bony metastases.

Radiography is also the first-line investigation for joints. Small, superficial joints can be visualised more closely with **ultrasound** for certain indications, and MRI is very good for detecting pathological changes.

Soft tissue is best visualised with ultrasound if the region is accessible. If not, MRI provides very good contrast for detecting pathologies in soft tissue.

Clinical insight

Remember the rule of twos for radiographs: two planes, two joints and two sides. With every radiograph the aim should be to show the bone in two planes. Include joints at both ends of the bones. Also, in some cases, and especially for children, obtain and compare radiographs of both limbs or both sides to help identify the underlying pathology.

2.1 Bony abnormalities

Many bony pathologies can be identified on plain radiographs. These include **fractures, arthritis** and **bony lesions**. Depending on the pathology suspected, further cross-sectional imaging with CT or MRI can then be used.

Stress fracture results when there is a mismatch between the strength of a bone strength and the stress placed upon it.

Fatigue fracture occurs when there is abnormal stress on normal bone.

Insufficiency fracture results from normal stress on abnormal bone.

Pathological fracture is a type of insufficiency fracture, but the term is reserved for fracture occurring at the site of a focal bony abnormality. Osteoporosis is the commonest cause of insufficiency fractures. Other diseases that cause bony abnormalities include Paget's disease, osteomalacia, osteogenesis imperfecta and bone tumours (benign or malignant, primary or secondary; see chapter 10, *Bony lesions*).

Characteristic	Variants
Site	• Proximal • Mid shaft • Distal • Metaphyseal • Diaphyseal
Pattern	• Transverse (segmental if two sequential transverse fractures are present with a floating segment between them)
	• Oblique
	• Spiral
	• Comminuted (variant subtype has triangular 'butterfly' fragment)
	• Avulsed
Displacement	• Translational (direction and degree of the distal fragment in relation to the proximal bone)

	• Angular (degree to the long axis of the proximal bone)
	  – Varus: angulation towards the midline
	  – Valgus: angulation away from the midline

	• Rotational (distal fragment is in a different plane to proximal bone)

Table 2.1 Description of fractures

Plain radiography

Carefully follow cortical outlines for any cortical break or bump and try to correlate it with the other plane. Some fractures may be present on a single plane only.

An **incomplete fracture** such as a greenstick fracture involves a single cortex in a single plane. A **complete fracture** involves both cortices. It is helpful to describe the fracture pattern accurately (**Table 2.1, Figures 2.1–2.4**).

Bony lesions disrupt the bone architecture (**Figure 2.5**; see p.201). Joint abnormalities caused by arthropathy are covered in detail on p.219.

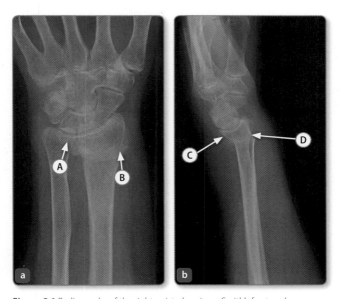

Figure 2.1 Radiographs of the right wrist, showing a Smith's fracture (see section 5.2, Distal forearm fractures). (a) Anteroposterior view showing translational displacement towards the ulnar side Ⓐ and overlap producing an area of increased density Ⓑ. (b) Lateral view showing dorsal angulation Ⓒ and an extra-articular transverse fracture Ⓓ of the distal radius.

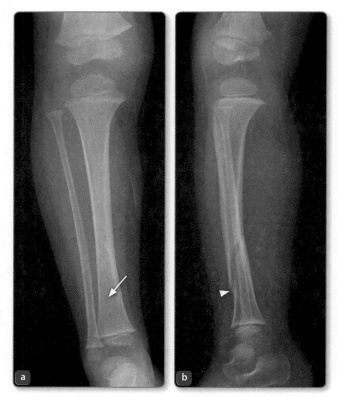

Figure 2.2 (a) Anteroposterior and (b) lateral radiographs of the right tibia and fibula, showing an oblique fracture of the distal tibial shaft, with minimal posterior displacement. The fracture line (arrow) is more difficult to see on the anteroposterior view, but the fracture gap (arrowhead) and displacement are evident on the lateral view.

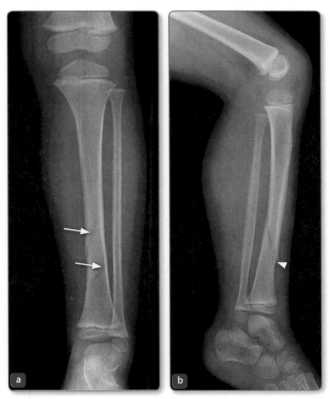

Figure 2.3 (a) Anteroposterior and (b) lateral radiographs of the left tibia and fibula, showing a spiral fracture (arrows) of the tibial shaft, with no significant displacement (arrowhead).

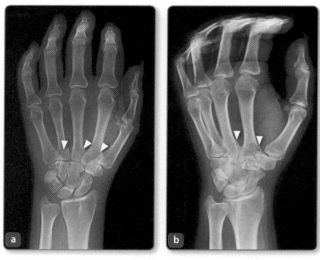

Figure 2.4 (a) Anteroposterior and (b) oblique radiographs of the left hand, showing transverse fractures (arrowheads) of the bases of the 2nd, 3rd and 4th metacarpals.

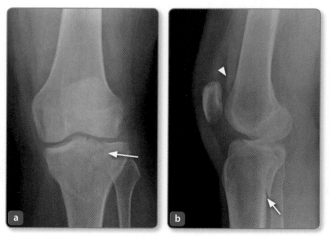

Figure 2.5 (a) Anteroposterior and (b) lateral radiographs of the right knee, showing minimal displacement caused by a lateral tibial plateau fracture (arrows). Lipohaemarthrosis (arrowhead) is visible on the lateral view (see section 7.2, Knee and tibial injuries).

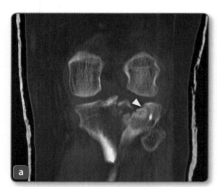

Figure 2.6 (a) Coronal and (b) sagittal computerised tomography of the right knee (in back slab; same patients as in Figure 2.5), showing the depressed (arrowhead) and displaced (arrow) fragments. These reconstructions were used to help plan surgery.

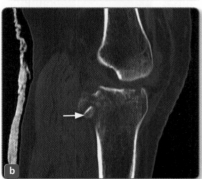

Computerised tomography

Computerised tomography is often used to detect occult fractures or to assess complex fractures to help in surgical planning. The use of sagittal and coronal reconstructions enables the fracture to be described with more accuracy than with just axial images (**Figure 2.6**).

Magnetic resonance imaging

Computerised tomography is better at evaluating the cortical break of a fracture, but MRI is very sensitive in detecting associated signs of bone marrow around the injury. Bone marrow appears as decreased signal on T1-weighted MRI or increased

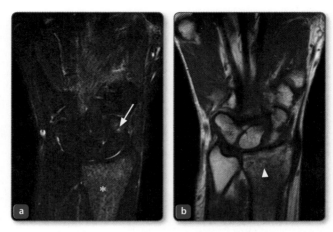

Figure 2.7 Coronal magnetic resonance imaging (MRI) of the right hand. (a) Short T1 inversion recovery (STIR) MRI shows marrow oedema in the distal radius (*), with a well-defined simple cyst in the scaphoid (arrow). (b) T1-weighted MRI shows low-signal fracture lines (arrowhead) in the distal radius, which are obscured on STIR MRI.

signal on short T1 inversion recovery (STIR) MRI. It is often masked on T2-weighted MRI because of surrounding hyperintense bone marrow oedema. Fracture lines appear as low signal on T1-weighted MRI (**Figure 2.7**).

Nuclear medicine
Pathologies that destroy bone increase bone turnover. The affected areas have increased uptake and are described as **hot** on **radionuclide imaging**. **Isotope bone scan** (**bone scintigraphy**) is used primarily to detect bony metastases (**Figures 2.8** and **2.9**). It can also help when looking for bony infection (particularly when a prosthesis or metalwork is present), which may be supplemented by a **leucocyte scan**. Bone scans were

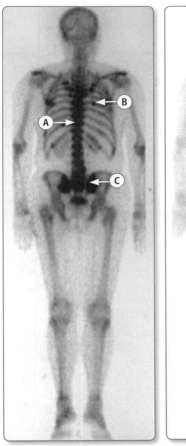

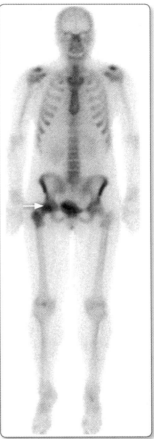

Figure 2.8 Isotope bone scan showing increased uptake in the spine Ⓐ, ribs Ⓑ and sacroiliac regions Ⓒ. These findings are consistent with widespread bony metastases.

Figure 2.9 Isotope bone scan showing isolated uptake in the right proximal femur (arrow). Further imaging confirmed a solitary bone metastasis.

historically used to detect occult fractures, but their lack of specificity means that CT or MRI has superseded them for this indication.

Multiple asymmetrical areas of increased uptake suggest bony metastases (**Figure 2.8**). Remember that lytic lesions such as myeloma may not elicit bone turnover; they therefore appear entirely normal on isotope bone scan. Areas of isolated focal uptake must be correlated with radiographs and sometimes MRI to confirm a solitary metastatic lesion (**Figure 2.9**).

Complete replacement of marrow by tumour can result in a uniform uptake known as a **superscan**. Maximal uptake is focused on the axial skeleton and proximal appendicular bones only, creating a headless or limbless appearance (**Figure 2.10**). Contrast this with a superscan caused by metabolic bone disease, which shows more uniform uptake, including in the distal appendicular extension, and intense calvarial uptake (**Figure 2.11**). Common metabolic bone diseases include renal osteodystrophy, hyperparathyroidism (typically secondary) and osteomalacia.

A **triple-phase bone scan** is needed for suspected osteomyelitis (**Table 2.2**) or infected metalwork. Infection is present when all three phases show increased, especially focal, uptake. If aseptic loosening is present (i.e. there is no infection), only the delayed phase show uptake in the surrounding bones, whereas the arterial and blood pool phases should be normal (see Figure 10.40).

Phase	What is represented	Osteomyelitis
1st: arterial	Dynamic phase showing blood flow to area	Focal hyperperfusion
2nd: blood pool	Extravasation of isotope into soft tissue	Focal hyperaemia
3rd: delayed	Bone uptake indicating turnover	Focal increase in bony uptake

Table 2.2 Phases of the triple-phase bone scan

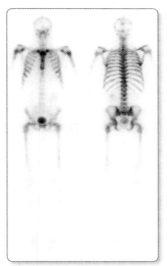

Figure 2.10 Isotope bone scan showing a so-called headless superscan indicating extensive marrow replacement by a metastatic tumour. There is intense uptake in the axial skeleton and proximal appendages.

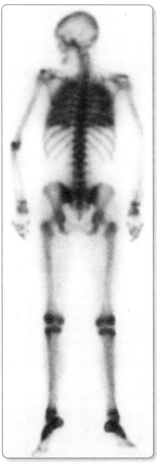

Figure 2.11 Isotope bone scan showing a superscan caused by the metabolic disease of secondary hyperparathyroidism. Compare the intense calvarial uptake and appendicular extension in this scan with Figure 2.10.

2.2 Tendon and ligament abnormalities

A **tendinopathy** is a disease of the tendon. Tendinopathy usually results from chronic overuse causing tendon deterioration without associated inflammation, a condition known as **tendinosis (Figure 2.12)**. **Tendinitis** is diagnosed when inflammation is present, more often in acute injuries. **Tenosynovitis** involves increased fluid in the tendon sheath (**Figure 2.13**).

Ultrasound

Ultrasound shows tendon pathologies very well. Focal areas of hypoechogenicity are areas of tendinosis. Sometimes, increased tendon size is the only sign of tendinosis. Increased power Doppler flow indicates vascularity, which should not be present within tendons, in keeping with tendinitis.

A defect in the tendon on ultrasound is a tear. If the defect is incomplete, then a **partial tear** is present (**Figure 2.14**). A **complete tear** shows loss of tendon fibrolinear continuity in the longitudinal axis (**Figure 2.15**).

> ### Clinical insight
>
> The main artefact in musculoskeletal ultrasound is **anisotropy**. Focal areas of hypoechogenicity occur if the ultrasound beam is not perpendicular to the structure examined. Slight obliquity of this angle of incidence can lead to marked changes. Because some musculoskeletal structures are curvilinear or oblique, this artefact cannot always be prevented. Hypoechoic areas that disappear on heel-to-toe rocking of the probe are not true pathological changes.

Magnetic resonance imaging

Tendinosis appears as focal irregular or diffuse intermediate signal intensity on T1-weighted and T2-weighted images. The tendon may show a diffuse or focal hypertrophy. Tears appear as areas of tissue loss. These areas may be replaced by fluid signal and therefore appear as high signal on T2-weighted images. However, in practice it can be difficult to distinguish severe tendinosis from a partial-thickness tear, and both can coexist. Ligament injuries are well shown on MRI.

- A **grade 1 sprain** shows normal thickness and signal intensity with associated perifascicular oedema, typically only external to the ligament.

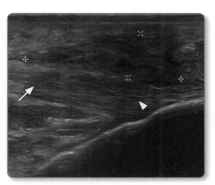

Figure 2.12 Longitudinal ultrasound of the patella tendon (arrow), showing areas of hypoechoicity (arrowhead) consistent with tendinopathy at its insertion on the tibial tuberosity. Infrapatellar bursitis is present superficially (+ and × mark the margins).

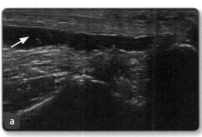

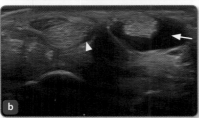

Figure 2.13 (a) Longitudinal and (b) transverse ultrasound of the finger, showing tenosynovitis of the flexor tendon. The tendon sheath contains an increased amount of fluid (arrow) compared with the normal small amount of fluid in the adjacent tendon sheath (arrowhead).

- A **grade 2 partial tear** has diffuse intrasubstance signal heterogeneity, with disrupted fibres and perifascicular oedema extending to between the bone and ligament.
- A **grade 3 full-thickness tear** has a completely disrupted ligament, often thickened and retracted, with an increased amount of surrounding oedema (**Figures 2.16–2.18**)

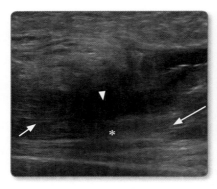

Figure 2.14 Longitudinal ultrasound of the quadriceps tendon, showing a partial-thickness tear (arrowhead) on the superficial surface. The intact remnant deep fibres (*) show continuity between the proximal (short arrow) and distal (long arrow) ends.

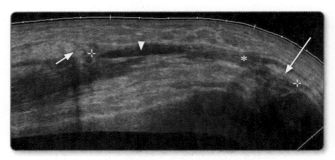

Figure 2.15 Longitudinal panoramic ultrasound of the quadriceps tendon, showing a full-thickness tear (arrowhead) with complete discontinuity (marked by +) between the proximal (short arrow) and distal (long arrow) ends. In the paratenon space is a hypoechoic haematoma (*).

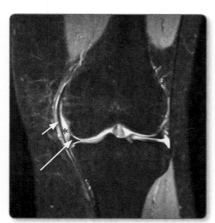

Figure 2.16 Coronal short T1 inversion recovery magnetic resonance imaging of the left knee, showing a grade 1 medial collateral ligament strain with thickening of the tendon (short arrow) and perifascicular fluid (*) surrounding the ligament and separating it from the medial meniscus (long arrow).

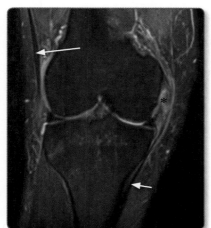

Figure 2.17 Coronal short T1 inversion recovery magnetic resonance imaging of the right knee, showing a grade 2 partial tear of the medial collateral ligament, with disrupted fibres (*) and intact distal ligament (short arrow). The iliotibial band laterally (long arrow) is normal.

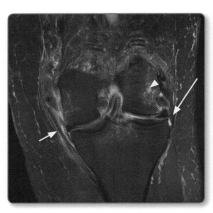

Figure 2.18 Coronal short T1 inversion recovery magnetic resonance imaging of the left knee, showing a grade 3 full-thickness tear (*) of the medial collateral ligament, with complete discontinuity to the distal, oedematous ligament (short arrow). Associated bruising (arrowhead) of the lateral femoral condylar bone is present. The lateral collateral ligament complex (long arrow) remains intact.

2.3 Muscular abnormalities

Muscular abnormalities other than traumatic tears can be broadly identified in three patterns: **muscular oedema**, **fatty infiltration** and **mass lesions**.

Ultrasound

Muscle strains can be divided into three grades of strain.

- **Grade 1 strains** do not show as muscular disruption. They may appear normal on ultrasound. Areas of focal or generalised increased echogenicity may be visible. Perifascial fluid may be present.
- **Grade 2 injuries** are partial tears of the musculature. Features include intrasubstance tears, seen as areas of hyperechogenicity, and disrupted **perimysial striae**. Perimysial striae are echogenic striae of the perimysium surrounding the low-echogenicity muscle fibres.
- **Grade 3 injuries** are full-thickness tears of the musculature. They are visible on ultrasound as complete discontinuity of muscle fibres, with an associated area of haematoma. The **clapper-in-bell sign** is a retracted echogenic muscular fragment in a hypoechoic haematoma.

Magnetic resonance imaging

Muscular tears are classified as shown in **Table 2.3**.

Muscular oedema

Areas of muscular oedema appear as increased signal on T2-weighted and STIR sequences (**Figure 2.19**). Signal changes

Grade	Disruption of muscle fibres (%)	Finding(s) on magnetic resonance imaging
1	< 10	• Hyperintense on short T1 inversion recovery • Feathery appearance if involving < 5% of muscle fibres
2	> 10 to < 50	• Features of oedema and haemorrhage at disrupted myotendinous junction
3	50–100	• Complete disruption of muscle continuity • Wavy tendon shape with retraction • Extensive oedema and haemorrhage

Table 2.3 Grading of muscular tears and their appearance on magnetic resonance imaging

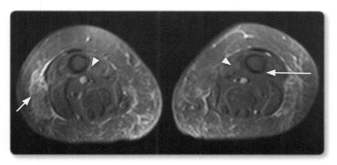

Figure 2.19 Short T1 inversion recovery magnetic resonance imaging of the thighs, showing increased signal in the vastus medialis bilaterally (arrowheads), consistent with myositis. Signal is also relatively increased in the rest of the right quadriceps, whereas the left remaining quadriceps is normal (long arrow). Non-specific subcutaneous oedema is present (short arrow).

may be focal, with ill-defined margins, or diffuse, affecting the whole muscle. Appearances are not specific to pathology, and many autoimmune conditions, such as polymyositis, can produce these changes.

Fatty infiltration

Fatty infiltration is caused by abnormal diffuse deposition of fat in a muscle. Many pathologies involving skeletal muscle can cause fatty infiltration. It is also seen in the chronic stages of muscle denervation. There tends to be associated muscle atrophy.

Mass lesions

This type of pattern shows a localised mass-like region with altered signal intensity on all sequences. Causes include neoplasm, intramuscular abscess, myonecrosis and myositis ossificans.

2.4 Soft tissue abnormalities

Various soft tissue abnormalities can be imaged. So-called **lumps** and **bumps** are common presentations. Radiological imaging can help clinicians understand the nature of these soft tissue lesions and decide how best to manage them. The presence of a **collection** or an **abscess** is also another important indication for soft tissue imaging. Sometimes a **haematoma** is present, in which case its age can be estimated.

Plain radiographs

Radiopaque soft tissue abnormalities are visible on radiographs. Two common groups, **soft tissue ossification** and **nodular and linear calcification**, and their differential diagnoses are listed in **Tables 2.4** and **2.5**.

Soft tissue swelling can also be shown on radiographs. Abscesses can also present with locules of free gas in the soft tissue (**Figure 2.23**).

Ultrasound

Ultrasound is primarily used to identify an abscess or collection, typically in a setting in which soft tissue infection such

Diagnosis	Note(s)
Soft tissue ossification	• Organised densities involving the cortex, the trabeculae or both
Heterotopic ossification (**Figure 2.20**)	• Typically calcifies 1 month after insult • Ossifies later • Most mature peripherally
Late myositis ossificans	• Ossification of muscles • Timing and zoning identical to in heterotopic ossification
Early myositis ossificans	• Amorphous calcification at < 1 month
Loose bodies	• Ossified round or oval masses in or around joints • Location can be confirmed on computerised tomography or magnetic resonance imaging
Haematoma	• Peripheral ossification in chronic cases
Sarcoma (osteosarcoma, synovial sarcoma or liposarcoma)	• Various sarcomas can ossify (see section 10.1, Bone tumours)

Table 2.4 Soft tissue ossification and common differential diagnoses

Diagnosis	Note(s)
Nodular or linear calcification	Structureless density in a globular or linear-to-curvilinear deposition
Phleboliths	Common small round calcifications of vessels with central lucency
Calcific tendinitis or bursitis (**Figure 2.21**)	Deposition of hydroxyapatite in tendons or bursa, typically after inflammation
Calcium pyrophosphate calcification	Deposition of calcium pyrophosphate dihydrate around joints (see p.219)
Haemangioma	Soft tissue mass with fat, vessels and phleboliths
Synovial osteochondromatosis	Multiple intra-articular densities visible on computerised tomography and magnetic resonance imaging (**Figure 2.22**)

Table 2.5 Nodular and linear calcification and common differential diagnoses

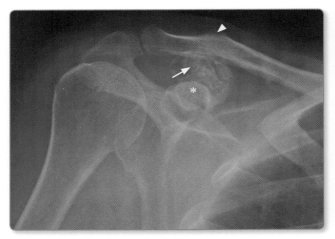

Figure 2.20 Anteroposterior radiograph of the right shoulder, showing heterotopic ossification (arrow) between the clavicle and the coracoid process (*). The ossification has probably occurred because of the now healed clavicle fracture (arrowhead).

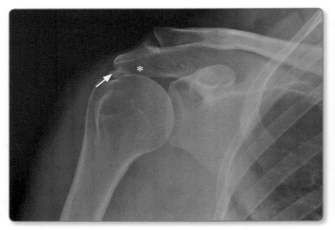

Figure 2.21 Anteroposterior radiograph of the right shoulder, showing nodular calcification (arrow) in the supraspinatus tendon in the subacromial space (*), consistent with underlying tendinopathy.

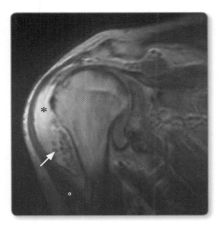

Figure 2.22 Coronal T2-weighted magnetic resonance imaging of the right shoulder, showing synovial chondromatosis (arrow) in the enlarged subacromial bursa, which is filled with fluid (*).

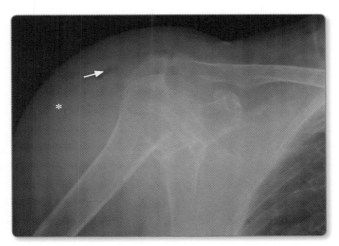

Figure 2.23 Anteroposterior radiograph of the right shoulder, showing gross soft tissue swelling (*) containing locules of free gas (arrow), consistent with a soft tissue abscess.

as cellulitis is diagnosed clinically. Diffuse thickening of subcutaneous tissue as a result of oedema is present in cellulitis, whereas the appearance of an actual abscess is more variable. Abscesses range from round and well defined to irregular (**Figure 2.24**) or lobulated. They can be anechoic to hyperechoic, often with internal echoes. Abscesses tend to show acoustic enhancement (**Figure 2.25**).

Soft tissue haematoma can also be well characterised on ultrasound. Chronic haematoma can mimic an abscess. Sometimes both may coexist (i.e. in an infected haematoma).

Ultrasound is also used to identify non-opaque foreign bodies, which can be well visualised. Depending on the irritability of the object, it can elicit surrounding granulomatous reaction as well as cause an abscess to develop (**Figure 2.26**).

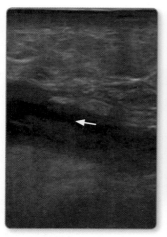

Figure 2.24 Ultrasound of the thigh, showing an abscess (arrow) in the subcutaneous tissue layer.

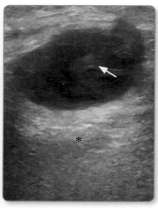

Figure 2.25 Ultrasound of soft tissue, showing a well-defined hypoechoic lesion with internal echogenicity (arrow) and acoustic enhancement (*), consistent with an abscess.

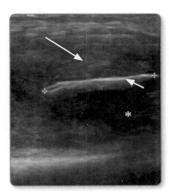

Figure 2.26 Ultrasound of the forearm, showing a foreign body (a wooden splinter, short arrow) in an anechoic abscess (*), with hypoechoic granulation tissue at the periphery (long arrow).

Computerised tomography

Computerised tomography is not the first-line investigation for soft tissue lesions. However, it can be used to accurately localise or further assess soft tissue pathology showing ossification (**Figure 2.27**) or calcification.

Magnetic resonance imaging

Complex abscesses, or deep-seated abscesses, which may be difficult to characterise on ultrasound, can be evaluated with MRI. Also, its relation and involvement with adjacent musculature and underlying bones can be identified (**Figure 2.28**).

Other soft tissue pathology, such as haematoma, is also well identified on MRI (**Figure 2.29**). Chronic haematoma has a low-signal rim because of the deposition of haemosiderin which has paramagnetic properties (**Figure 2.30**). The signal within varies depending on the age of the haematoma (**Table 2.6**).

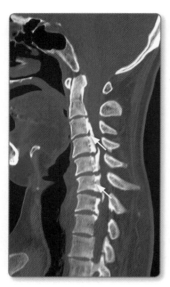

Figure 2.27 Sagittal computerised tomography of the cervical spine, showing an ossifying posterior longitudinal ligament (arrows).

Phase	No. of days	T1-weighted	T2-weighted	Pathology
Hyperacute	< 1	Isointense/low	High	Intracellular oxyhaemoglobin
Acute	1–3	Low	Low	Intracellular deoxyhaemoglobin
Early subacute	3–7	High	Low	Intracellular haemoglobin
Late subacute	7–14	High	High	Extracellular haemoglobin
Chronic	> 14	Low	Low	Haemosiderin

Table 2.6 Signal intensities of haematoma according to age and magnetic resonance imaging sequence

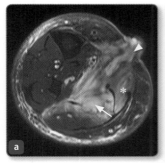

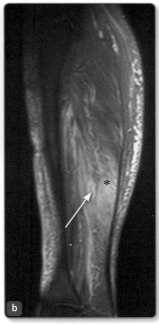

Figure 2.28 (a) Axial and (b) sagittal short T1 inversion recovery magnetic resonance imaging of the left leg, showing an abscess (arrow) communicating with a sinus tract (arrowhead). Local muscular oedema (stars) is present in the surrounding tissue, but the underlying bones remain normal.

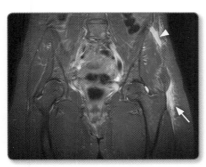

Figure 2.29 Coronal short T1 inversion recovery magnetic resonance imaging of the pelvis, showing haematoma between the superficial subcutaneous layer and the deeper musculature and bone (arrow). The haematoma also extends proximally (arrowhead).

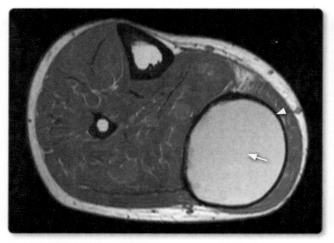

Figure 2.30 Axial T2-weighted magnetic resonance imaging of the left calf, showing chronic haematoma with high-signal fluid (arrow) and low-signal haemosiderin deposition in the well-defined walls (arrowhead).

Shoulder

3.1 Key anatomy

The shoulder girdle is formed by the clavicle, the scapula and the head of the humerus (**Figure 3.1**). The coracoid process projects anteriorly from the scapula and is an important attachment point for various muscles and ligaments. The glenoid fossa is attached to the glenoid labrum, a fibrocartilaginous ring that deepens the glenoid cavity (see p.57). The rotator cuff comprises the supraspinatus, infraspinatus, teres minor and subscapularis muscles. The subscapularis arises from the scapula to attach to the tuberosities.

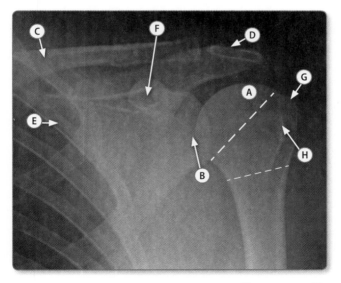

Figure 3.1 Anteroposterior radiograph of the left shoulder. (A) Humeral head, (B) glenoid fossa, (C) clavicle, (D) acromion process, (E) rib, (F) coracoid process, (G) greater tuberosity, (H) lesser tuberosity. The position of the anatomical neck (thick dashed line) and the surgical neck (thin dashed line) of the humerus are shown.

Imaging points

- Anteroposterior radiography is used to assess the shoulder girdle. Additionally, either a lateral scapular (also known as a Y view, **Figure 3.2**) or an axial view through the armpit (**Figure 3.3**) is often included.
- In children and adolescents, the proximal epiphyseal line is cone-shaped (**Figure 3.4**). Do not mistake this line for a fracture.
- Which other imaging modality to use depends on the clinical situation.
    - **Computerised tomography** is best for occult or complex fractures; scans are helpful in surgical planning.
    - **Ultrasound** is an extremely sensitive technique for assessing the rotator cuff.
    - **Magnetic resonance imaging** (MRI) is the preferred method for imaging the rest of the muscles, ligaments and soft tissues (**Figures 3.5–3.7**), and MRI arthrograms can be done to assess labral pathology.

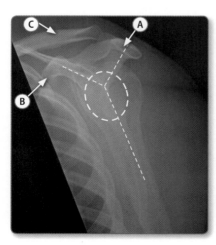

Figure 3.2 Lateral scapular radiograph of the left shoulder. The humeral head normally projects over the glenoid fossa (thick dashed line), and the centre of the glenoid fossa lies roughly at the centre of the Y (thin dashed line). If the humeral head does not project over the glenoid fossa, the glenohumeral joint is dislocated. The Y shape is formed by the spine of the scapula, which continues as the acromion process (A), the coracoid process (B) and the blade of the scapula. (C) Clavicle.

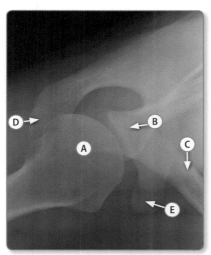

Figure 3.3 Axial radiograph of the right shoulder. The humeral head Ⓐ can clearly be seen articulating with the glenoid fossa Ⓑ. The imaging plate is placed horizontally under the armpit, and the X-ray beam is focused onto the imaging plate from above. This view requires abduction of the shoulder, which the patient may find difficult. Ⓒ Clavicle, Ⓓ acromion process, Ⓔ coracoid process.

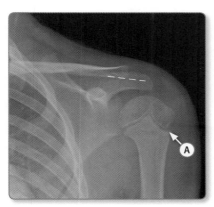

Figure 3.4 Anteroposterior radiograph of the left shoulder of a child. The epiphyseal line Ⓐ is a normal finding and should not be confused with a fracture. The inferior margin of the acromion aligns with the inferior margin of the clavicle (dashed line).

- The inferior margin of the acromion should align with the inferior margin of the clavicle with which it articulates (**Figure 3.1**). If the line between the inferior margin of the acromion and the inferior margin of the clavicle is disrupted, suspect an acromioclavicular joint injury.

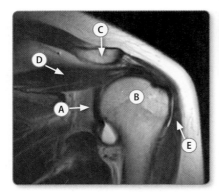

Figure 3.5 Coronal T2-weighted MRI of the left shoulder. (A) Glenoid fossa, (B) humeral head, (C) acromion process, (D) supraspinatus, (E) deltoid.

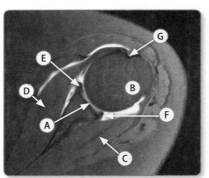

Figure 3.6 Axial T2-weighted MRI of the left shoulder. (A) Glenoid fossa, (B) humeral head, (C) infraspinatus, (D) subscapularis, (E) anterior glenoid labrum, (F) posterior glenoid labrum, (G) intertubercular groove containing the long head of the biceps.

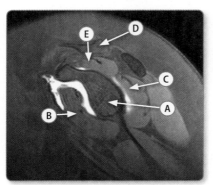

Figure 3.7 Sagittal T2-weighted MRI of the left shoulder. (A) Glenoid fossa, (B) subscapularis, (C) infraspinatus, (D) acromion process, (E) supraspinatus.

- The anatomical neck of the humerus is just below the head of the humerus, between it and the greater and lesser tuberosities (**Figure 3.1**). The surgical neck is further down from the anatomical neck, between the expanded proximal end of the humerus and the shaft (**Figure 3.1**). The surgical neck is clinically important in proximal humeral fractures.

3.2 Shoulder dislocations

A shoulder dislocation is complete loss of articulation between the humeral head and the glenoid fossa of the scapula. Dislocations are anterior, posterior or inferior, depending on the location of the dislocated humeral head with respect to the glenoid fossa. After a shoulder dislocation, the joint capsule becomes lax and predisposed to instability.

Key facts
- About 95% of shoulder dislocations are anterior and are secondary to forced abduction, external rotation and extension (**Figure 3.8**).
- About 5% of shoulder dislocations are posterior and associated with electric shock or seizure (**Figure 3.9**).
- Inferior dislocations, also known as luxatio erecta, are very rare (**Figure 3.10**). However, this type of shoulder dislocation is easy to diagnose clinically, because the patient presents with the arm raised in a fixed position above the head.

Radiological findings

Radiography Shoulder dislocations involve complete loss of congruity between the humeral head and the glenoid fossa. The humeral head is displaced anteriorly (below the coracoid process), posteriorly or inferiorly relative to the glenoid fossa. Bones may be injured as the humeral head impacts against the glenoid fossa at the time of dislocation. See section 3.6, Glenoid labral pathology, for associated pathological changes in the glenoid labrum.
- **A Hill–Sachs lesion** involves impaction of the posterosuperior humeral head (**Figure 3.11**).

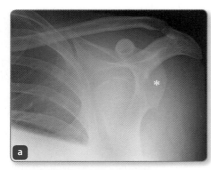

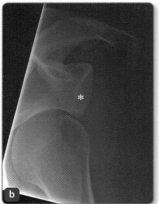

Figure 3.8 (a) Anteroposterior and (b) oblique radiographs of the left shoulder, showing anterior dislocation of the humeral head. The oblique view confirms complete loss of congruity with the glenoid fossa (*).

- **A bony Bankart lesion** involves anteroinferior fracture of the bony glenoid fossa (see section 3.6 for appearances on MRI).

Key imaging findings
- There is loss of articulation.
- A Hills–Sachs or Bankart lesion is visible.
- In an anterior dislocation, the humeral head projects below the coracoid process.

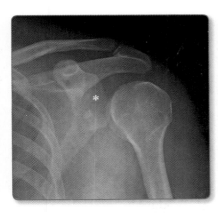

Figure 3.9
Anteroposterior radiograph of the left shoulder, showing posterior dislocation of the humeral head. The loss of overlap between the humeral head and the glenoid fossa (*) result in the characteristic light bulb sign. An axial or lateral Y view can help confirm the diagnosis.

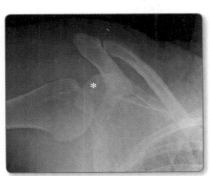

Figure 3.10
Anteroposterior radiograph of the right shoulder, showing inferior dislocation of the humeral head. The humeral head lies low relative to the glenoid fossa (*).

- In a posterior dislocation, the head and neck of the humerus resemble a light bulb on anteroposterior radiographs.

Treatment

Shoulder dislocations usually need to be reduced by a medical professional. However, recurrent dislocations may self-reduce because the joint capsule is lax. Surgical management may be needed for long-term stabilisation.

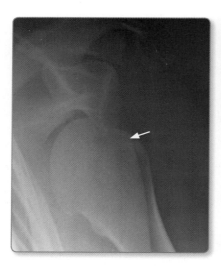

Figure 3.11
Anteroposterior radiograph of the left shoulder, showing anterior dislocation of the humeral head. The posterosuperior deformity is consistent with a Hill–Sachs lesion (arrow).

3.3 Acromioclavicular joint and clavicle injuries

Injuries to the acromioclavicular joint and clavicle are usually caused by a direct blow. Pain is commonly localised, with the patient able to pinpoint the area of maximal tenderness over the joint or the fracture line.

Key facts

- The normal acromioclavicular joint distance is ≤ 8 mm. A distance of > 8 mm between acromion and clavicle indicates a ruptured acromioclavicular ligament.
- The inferior margins of the clavicle and the acromion should align (**Figure 3.7**). A total dislocation is present if the inferior margin of the clavicle is higher than the superior margin of the acromion (**Figure 3.12**).
- Clavicular fractures can occur in isolation, without injury to the acromion (**Figure 3.13**).

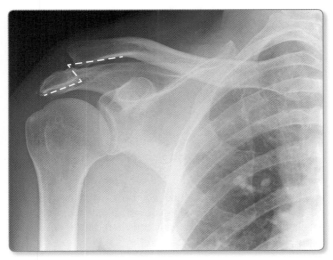

Figure 3.12 Anteroposterior radiograph of the right shoulder, showing complete dislocation of the end of the lateral clavicle from the acromion. This injury causes the bones to resemble steps (dashed white line). A type 4 Rockwood dislocation is shown.

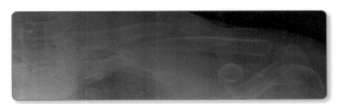

Figure 3.13 Anteroposterior radiograph of the left clavicle, demonstrating clavicular mid-shaft fracture with complete translational displacement and shortening. The acromion is intact.

Radiological findings

Radiography A plain anteroposterior radiograph is best for viewing the acromioclavicular joint and assessing pathological changes associated with acute injuries in this region.

Injuries are classified according to acromioclavicular alignment and distance (**Table 3.1**). Assess the alignment between the undersurfaces of the acromion and the clavicle to identify subluxations and dislocations. Measure the acromioclavicular distance to assess the joint for sprain, subluxation and dislocation.

Key imaging findings
- The inferior surfaces of the acromion and the clavicle do not align.
- The lateral end of the clavicle moves cranially in acromioclavicular subluxations and dislocations.

Treatment
Injuries to the acromioclavicular joint and clavicle are managed conservatively. A shoulder sling is used for mild injuries. Surgical fixation and reconstruction is considered for more severe injuries (Rockwood type 4 or above).

3.4 Proximal humeral fractures

Fractures of the proximal humerus are commonly found in elderly patients and in patients with osteoporosis after a fall onto an outstretched hand.

Type	Injury	Radiographic findings
1	Mild sprain	Unremarkable radiograph
2	Moderate sprain	Increased acromioclavicular distance secondary to tears of the acromioclavicular ligaments
3	Severe sprain	Acromioclavicular and coracoclavicular distances increased because of tears of the acromioclavicular and corocaclavicular ligaments
4	Total dislocation	Lateral end of the clavicle superoposteriorly displaced into the trapezial fascia
5	Total dislocation	Lateral end of the clavicle displaced into the neck
6	Total dislocation	Lateral end of the clavicle displaced inferiorly into the subacromial or subcoracoid space

Table 3.1 Rockwood radiographic classification of acromioclavicular joint and clavicle injuries

Key fact
- Proximal humeral fractures often occur in patients with weakened bones.

Radiological findings

Radiography Fractures of the proximal humerus are identified by cortical disruption and displacement of fracture fragments.

Classification is based on the type of displacement and the number of fracture fragments. The four segments considered in the Neer classification system are the anatomical neck, the surgical neck, the greater tuberosity and the lesser tuberosity. Displacement of fragments is defined as > 1 cm separation of fracture fragments and > 45° increase in angulation.

Key imaging finding
- Pay particular attention to the displacement and number of fracture fragments. Management of proximal humeral fractures depends on classification.

Treatment
Fractures of the proximal humerus are treated according to their grade (**Table 3.2**).

Grade	Description	Treatment
One-part fracture	No displaced fragments, regardless of comminution (**Figure 3.14**)	Conservative: sling
Two-part fracture	One displaced fragment	Conservative: closed reduction
Three-part fracture	Two displaced fragments, with one intact tuberosity	Conservative: closed reduction
Four-part fracture	Three displaced fragments (**Figure 3.15**)	Surgical reduction with optional humeral head prosthesis

Table 3.2 Classification and treatment of fractures of the proximal humerus

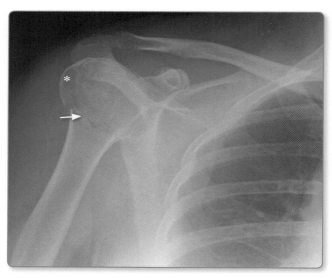

Figure 3.14 Anteroposterior radiograph of the right shoulder, showing a proximal humeral fracture traversing the surgical neck (arrow) and involving the greater tuberosity (*). The fracture is undisplaced in the Neer classification.

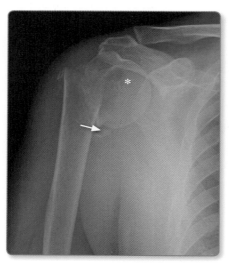

Figure 3.15 Anteroposterior radiograph of the right shoulder, demonstrating a 3-part fracture. Note the anteriorly displaced lesser tuberosity (arrow) below the humeral head (*) with intact greater tuberosity.

3.5 Rotator cuff pathology

The rotator cuff consists of the supraspinatus, infraspinatus, teres minor and subscapularis muscles. It provides dynamic stability to the shoulder joint.

The rotator cuff is a common source of pain caused by impingement syndrome. In this condition, the acromion impinges on the supraspinatus and overlying subacromial bursa. Impingement syndrome may develop as a result of trauma or have no specific cause.

Key facts

- Pathological changes in the rotator cuff typically present with painful shoulder. The pain may radiate to the arm and restrict lifting movements.
- Tendons can show tendinopathy and sometimes partial- or full-thickness tears.
- Acromioclavicular joint arthropathy can also contribute to impingement syndrome.

Radiological findings

Radiography A curved or hooked shape may predispose the acromion to impingement. The acromiohumeral distance may be reduced. Soft tissue calcification indicates calcific tendonitis.

Ultrasound Tendinopathy can be present, with calcific deposits in chronic cases. These calcific deposits often cast anechoic shadows (**Figure 3.16**). The subacromial bursa is often thickened because of the increased amount of fluid it contains (**Figure 3.16**). Partial- or full-thickness tears may be present (**Figure 3.17a**).

Magnetic resonance imaging Features are similar to those of ultrasound scans (**Figure 3.17b**). MRI provides information about chronicity, including wasting of the muscle belly, and is particularly useful in patients with markedly restricted shoulder movement.

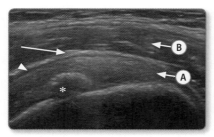

Figure 3.16 Ultrasound longitudinal view of the supraspinatus tendon (A). The thickened subacromial bursa (long arrow) contains an increased amount of bursal fluid (arrowhead). The bursa lies deep to the deltoid muscle (B). In the tendon is a calcific deposit (*) showing acoustic shadowing.

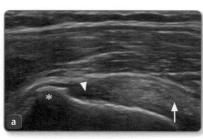

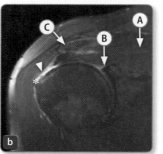

Figure 3.17 (a) Ultrasound longitudinal view and (b) coronal magnetic resonance imaging (MRI, short T1 inversion recovery) of the right supraspinatus tendon (A), showing a discontinuity in the tendon, in keeping with a full-thickness tear (arrowhead) at its insertion on the greater tuberosity (*). The glenoid labrum (B) and acromion (C) are visible on MRI.

Key imaging findings

- Partial-thickness tears of the supraspinatus can be superficial (on the bursal surface), deep (on the articular surface) or intrasubstance.

- Beware of anisotropy on ultrasound. Anisotropy caused by the curvature of the tendons can be a false positive for a tear.
- Doppler flow may sometimes be increased at calcific deposits (in cases of calcific tendinitis) or in bursal walls (in cases of bursitis).

Treatment

Most cases of rotator cuff pathology are managed conservatively. Some cases may need cortisone injection into the subacromial bursa, which can be done using anatomical landmarks or under ultrasound guidance. Subacromial decompression (for impingement syndrome) or cuff repair (for full-thickness tears) are needed in specific cases.

3.6 Glenoid labral pathology

The glenoid labrum is commonly torn or avulsed when excessive force is applied to the glenohumeral joint. A superior labral anterior–posterior (SLAP) is a common injury in athletes whose sport involves throwing.

Key facts

- The **Bankart lesion** is an anteroinferior labral tear commonly associated with anterior dislocation, which is usually recurrent. It is a bony Bankart lesion if the bony component is avulsed with the labrum (**Figure 3.18**). A reverse Bankart lesion is a posterior labral tear with posterior dislocations. Variant Bankart lesions (**Table 3.3**) include the Perthes lesion (**Figure 3.19**).
- Many types of **SLAP lesion** have been described. However, the four classic types are:
  - type 1, partial tear or fraying of labrum
  - type 2, the commonest type, with associated instability of the biceps anchor (**Figure 3.20**)
  - type 3, the so-called bucket handle type of tear, with intact labrum
  - type 4, with the labral tear extending into the long head of the biceps tendon

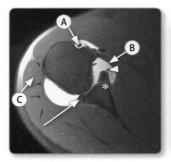

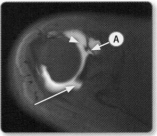

Figure 3.18 Axial T1-weighted magnetic resonance imaging of the left shoulder with fat saturation, showing a Bankart lesion (arrowhead) with a bony component (*). The posterior inferior labrum is intact (long arrow). (A) Long head of biceps tendon, (B) subscapularis muscle, (C) deltoid muscle.

Figure 3.19 Axial T1-weighted magnetic resonance imaging of the left shoulder with fat saturation, showing a Perthes lesion (a variant Bankart lesion). The anterior labrum is avulsed (arrowhead), and there is associated stripping of the periosteal sleeve (A). The posterior labrum (long arrow) remains intact.

Lesion	Abbreviation
Perthes lesion: labral avulsion with intact but stripped periosteum	–
Anterior labral periosteal sleeve avulsion: intact anterior periosteum with medially displaced labrum	ALPSA
Glenolabral articular disruption with associated glenoid chondral defect	GLAD
Humeral avulsion of the glenohumeral ligament, involving inferior glenohumeral ligament avulsion	HAGL

Table 3.3 Variant Bankart lesions

Radiological findings

Magnetic resonance imaging Diagnosis of labral tears is based on abnormalities in signal intensity, shape and displacement of the labrum. Use of an MRI arthrogram with intra-articular gadolinium contrast injection improves accuracy. The abducted

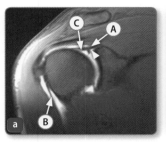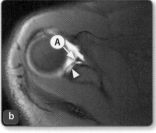

Figure 3.20 Coronal and axial T1-weighted magnetic resonance imaging of the right shoulder with fat saturation, showing a type 2 superior labral anterior–posterior tear. Contrast is tracking (arrowheads) beneath the superior labrum Ⓐ from anterior to posterior. Ⓑ Biceps, Ⓒ biceps anchor.

and externally rotated position can help make labral tears more conspicuous on MRI.

Key imaging findings

- Contrast tracking beneath the labrum and away from the glenoid fossa is more likely to indicate a tear than contrast tracking along the glenoid contour, which may indicate a sublabral recess.
- The site of the labral tear can be used to differentiate tears. SLAP tears are in the superior labrum, whereas Bankart lesions are in the anteroinferior labrum.
- Secondary signs include paralabral cysts, periosteal stripping and associated bone injuries (e.g. a Hill–Sachs lesion).

Treatment

Specialist shoulder orthopaedic management is usually needed for anatomic arthroscopic repair for patients able to undergo surgery.

4.1 Key anatomy

The elbow is a hinge joint consisting of the humerus, the ulna and the radius. The trochlea articulates with the coronoid process and the olecranon. The capitellum articulates with the radial head. The proximal radioulnar pivot joint forms the 3rd elbow articulation, between the radial head and the radial notch of the ulna. This joint acts as a pivot for supination and pronation of the forearm.

The common flexor tendon arises from the medial epicondyle, and the common extensor tendon arises from the lateral epicondyle. The ulnar nerve passes through the cubital channel on the posterior surface of the medial condyle. The distal biceps tendon is lateral to the brachial vessels.

Imaging points

- Radiography remains the first-line imaging modality. Orthogonal anteroposterior radiography (**Figure 4.1**) and lateral radiography (**Figure 4.2**) are used in the routine assessment of the elbow.
- On both anteroposterior and lateral radiographs, the radiocapitellar line drawn through the mid radial neck must always pass through the capitellum (**Figure 4.1**).
- The anterior humeral line must pass through the middle third of the capitellum. Failure to do so suggests a displaced supracondylar fracture.
- The anterior fat pad is visible as a slim radiolucent area anteriorly (**Figure 4.2**). However, the posterior fat pad is never seen in a normal elbow.
- A number of ossification centres are visible in radiographs of children, depending on their age (**Table 4.1**).
- Computerised tomography is used primarily for presurgical planning for complex fracture patterns or for the detection of loose bodies. Computerised tomography may also help in the detection of occult fractures.

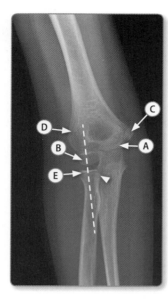

Figure 4.1 Anteroposterior radiograph of the right elbow, showing the trochlea (A), capitellum (B) and medial epicondyle (C). The lateral epicondyle ossification centre (which would be at point (D)) is not yet visible in this radiograph from a 9-year-old child. The radial head (E) articulates at the proximal radioulnar joint (arrowhead). The radiocapitellar line (dashed) crosses the capitellum.

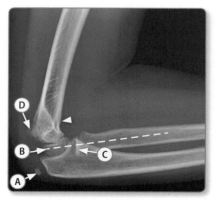

Figure 4.2 Lateral radiograph of the right elbow, showing the olecranon (A), capitellum (B) and radial head (C). The radiocapitellar line (dashed) crosses the capitellum. The medial epicondyle (D) is visible. A slim anterior fat pad (arrowhead) is present.

Ossification centre	Approximate age (range) at which ossification centre appears (years)
Capitellum	1 (1–2)
Radial head	3 (2–4)
Internal (medial) epicondyle	5 (4–6)
Trochlea	8 (7–11)
Olecranon	9 (9–11)
External (lateral) epicondyle	11 (10–11)

Table 4.1 Ossification centres of the elbow in children

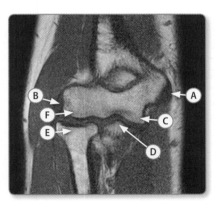

Figure 4.3 Coronal T1-weighted magnetic resonance imaging of the right elbow, showing the common flexor (A) and extensor (B) tendon origins, as well as bony structures including the trochlea (C), coronoid process (D), radial head (E) and capitellum (F).

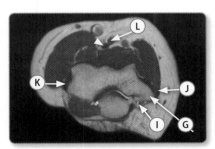

Figure 4.4 Axial T2-weighted magnetic resonance imaging of the right elbow, showing the common flexor (J) and extensor (K) tendon origins. Posterior to the medial epicondyle (G) lies the ulna nerve (I) within the cubital channel. The biceps tendon (L) is seen lateral to brachial artery (arrowhead).

Clinical insight

If the olecranon ossification centre is visible but the medial (internal) epicondyle is not, this indicates an avulsion injury of the medial epicondyle. The epicondyle has been displaced; it is likely to be overlapping other bones.

- Magnetic resonance imaging (MRI) is good for visualising soft tissue, such as the common flexor and extensor tendon origins, the ulnar nerve and the distal biceps tendon (**Figures 4.3** and **4.4**).

4.2 Elbow trauma

The elbow is an important site for traumatic injuries as well as common chronic disorders (e.g. tennis elbow). Both fractures and dislocations occur at the elbow. When interpreting elbow radiographs, consider the patient's age; specific injuries tend to occur in certain age groups.

The following eponymous fractures are uncommon but often discussed. The Monteggia fracture is a fracture of the ulna and a dislocation of the radial head (**Figure 4.5**). The Galeazzi fracture is a fracture of the radial shaft (usually at the junction of the middle and distal third), with associated subluxation or dislocation of the distal radioulnar joint (**Figure 4.6**).

Key facts

- An elevated anterior fat pad (the sail sign) and the presence of a posterior fat pad (always abnormal) indicates a haemarthrosis and an intra-articular elbow fracture (**Figure 4.7**). Elevated fat pads may be the only radiographic finding in an occult fracture of the elbow.
- Elbow fractures in infants and young children are most commonly supracondylar (**Figure 4.8**). Many supracondylar fractures are radiographically occult.
- The most common elbow fractures in adults involve the radial head or neck (**Figure 4.7**). Any bone or bony process in the elbow (e.g. the coronoid process, olecranon or trochlea) can fracture.

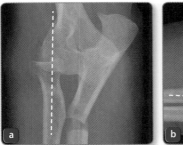
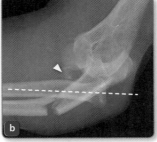

Figure 4.5 (a) Anteroposterior and (b) lateral radiographs of the right elbow, showing a Monteggia fracture. Dislocation of the ulna causes dislocation of the radial head, so that the radiocapitellar line (dashed) no longer crosses the capitellum. An associated fragment (arrowhead) was confirmed as a coronoid process fracture on computerised tomography (not shown).

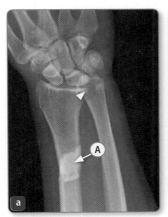
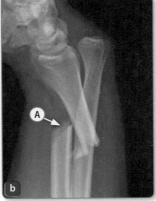

Figure 4.6 (a) Anteroposterior and (b) lateral radiographs of left wrist showing a Galeazzi fracture of the distal third of the radial shaft Ⓐ, with overlapping areas of increased opacity. There is disruption of the distal radioulnar joint (arrowhead) with a dislocated distal ulna.

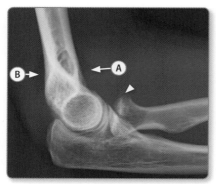

Figure 4.7 Lateral radiograph of the left elbow, showing the sail sign of an elevated anterior fat pad (A) and the presence of a posterior fat pad (B). These findings indicate haemarthrosis caused by a radial head fracture (arrowhead).

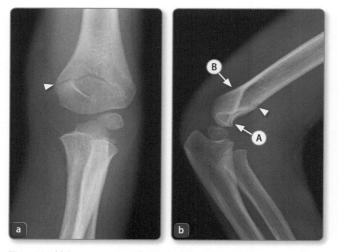

Figure 4.8 (a) Anteroposterior radiograph of the left elbow, showing a supracondylar fracture (arrowhead) in a child. (b) A lateral radiograph shows a subtle undisplaced cortical break (arrowhead) in this undisplaced fracture, but the underlying sail sign (A) and presence of a posterior fat pad (B) should alert the clinician to look for a supracondylar fracture.

Radiological findings

Radiography Loss of cortical integrity, radiolucent lines and displaced bone fragments are seen in fractures of the elbow. Elbow dislocations involve loss of articulation between the radial head and the capitellum of the humerus (radial head dislocation; **Figure 4.5**), disassociation of the proximal ulna from the trochlea of the humerus (complete elbow dislocation), or both.

Key imaging findings

- A step in the cortex or a radiolucent line is seen in displaced fractures.
- In adults, the radiocapitellar line should always intersect the radial head and the capitellum (**Figures 4.1** and **4.2**). Misalignment indicates subluxation or dislocation of the radial head (**Figure 4.5**).

Treatment

Most simple fractures are treated by reduction and immobilisation. Complex injuries may need open reduction and internal fixation.

4.3 Epicondylitis

Epicondylitis is inflammation of the common extensor or flexor tendon of the elbow.

Key facts

- Lateral epicondylitis involving the common extensor tendon origin is known as tennis elbow and accounts for 80% of cases of epicondylitis.
- Lateral epicondylitis is typically an overuse injury caused by repetitive extension or flexion of the elbow.
- Imaging is reserved for cases refractory to non-surgical management.

Radiological findings

Ultrasound   A focal hypoechoic area or thickening (**Figure 4.9**) can be seen deep in the common tendon origin. There may be active Doppler flow, which indicates active inflammation. A minority of cases of epicondylitis involve discrete partial- or full-thickness tears.

Magnetic resonance imaging   There is increased signal return at the common tendon origin on T2-weighted and short T1 inversion recovery sequences. Underlying bone marrow oedema may be visible. Focal linear fluid signal in the tendon indicates a tear (**Figure 4.10**).

Key imaging findings
- The common extensor or flexor tendon origin has a typical tendinopathic appearance.
- It is important to detect any associated partial- or full-thickness tears.

Treatment
Over 90% of cases of epicondylitis resolve in 4–6 weeks with simple oral analgesia, splints and physiotherapy. Corticosteroid

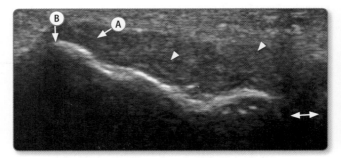

Figure 4.9 Longitudinal ultrasound view of the elbow, showing a thickened hypoechoic common extensor tendon (A) arising from the lateral epicondyle (B) proximal to the elbow joint (double arrows). Doppler flow is present in the inflamed tendon (arrowheads).

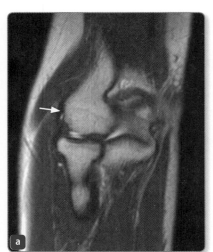

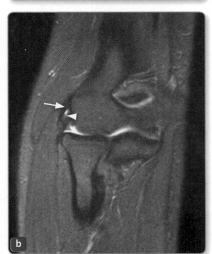

Figure 4.10 (a) Coronal T2-weighted and (b) short T1 inversion recovery (STIR) magnetic resonance imaging of the right elbow. The thickened common extensor tendon (arrows), with focal increased fluid signal (arrowheads), is consistent with a partial-thickness tear. These features are clearer in the STIR image.

injections can be beneficial in recalcitrant cases. Surgical tendon release can help in non-responsive cases.

4.4 Distal biceps tendon rupture

The distal biceps tendon may rupture from its insertion on the radial tuberosity. The rupture usually presents as a painful, swollen elbow after a traumatic event. If a full-thickness tear is confirmed, identifying the site of proximal tendon retraction can help in surgical fixation.

Key facts

- Distal biceps tendon rupture usually occurs in middle-aged men. The injury presents with a sudden painful tearing sensation over the antecubital fossa.
- The mechanism of injury usually involves sudden extension when the forearm is flexed or supinated.

Radiological findings

Ultrasound Features of a tendon rupture are present, either a partial-thickness tear or a complete tear (**Figure 4.11**) with varying degrees of tendon retraction. Associated surrounding hypoechoic fluid suggesting oedema or haemorrhage is often seen.

Magnetic resonance imaging Partial-thickness tears retain some form of continuity, with surrounding high signal intensity on T2-weighted imaging (**Figure 4.12**). Full-thickness tears show tendinous discontinuity with retraction.

Treatment

Management of distal biceps tendon rupture depends on

> **Clinical insight**
>
> Patients tend to present with the so-called Popeye sign: a biceps muscle bunched-up from tendon retraction.

> **Clinical insight**
>
> In imaging studies, the brachial artery is a good landmark to use when identifying the distal biceps tendon. The tendon runs parallel to the artery.

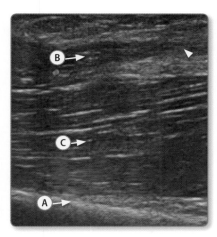

Figure 4.11 Longitudinal ultrasound view of the distal humerus (A), showing proximal retraction of the distal biceps tendon (B) caused by a full-thickness tear. An empty tendon sheath is visible distally (arrowhead). The underlying brachialis (C) is normal.

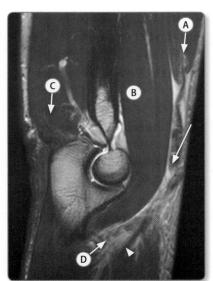

Figure 4.12 Sagittal T2-weighted magnetic resonance imaging of the right elbow, showing the biceps belly (A) and retraction of the proximal tendon (long arrow) caused by a partial-thickness tear. The distal tendon (D) is ill defined before the insertion (not shown). The brachial artery (arrowhead) is adjacent. (B) Underlying normal brachialis, (C) triceps muscle.

the degree of tear, the amount of remnant function and the age of the injury. Surgery is indicated for patients unable to tolerate loss of supination strength with non-operative treatment.

Wrist and hand

5.1 Key anatomy

The wrist is formed by the articulation of the radius and ulna with the carpal bones (**Figures 5.1** and **5.2**). The proximal carpal row comprises the scaphoid, lunate, triquetrum and pisiform. The distal carpal row consists of the trapezium, trapezoid, capitate and hamate (from lateral to medial). The carpal bones are not flat but are arranged in an arch spanned by a ligament called the flexor retinaculum. Thus the carpal bones form a space called the carpal tunnel (**Figure 5.3**).

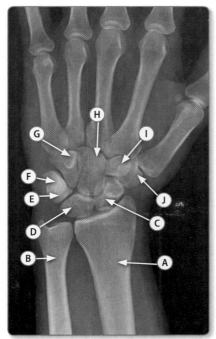

Figure 5.1
Anteroposterior radiograph of the left wrist. (A) Radius, (B) ulna, (C) scaphoid, (D) lunate, (E) triquetrum, (F) pisiform, (G) hamate, (H) capitate, (I) trapezoid, (J) trapezium.

The relation of the distal ulna to the distal radius is the ulnar variance. Ulnar variance is neutral when the ulna and the radius end at the same level, independent of the length of the styloid process. Ulnar variance is positive if the ulna projects distal to the radius. It is negative if the ulna projects proximal to the radius.

Imaging points

- Ultrasound shows pathological changes in tendons and is sensitive for joint synovitis.
- On a normal lateral radiograph of the wrist, the distal radius, lunate and capitate align. Imagine a cup (the lunate) sitting on a saucer (the radius) containing an apple (the capitate) (**Figure 5.2**).
- The articular end of the radius usually tilts in a volar direction by about 10°. However, a tilt of up to 20° may also be normal.
- The extensor tendons run deep to the extensor retinaculum. These tendons are divided into six compartments (**Figure 5.4**). The tendons in each compartment are listed in **Table 5.1**.

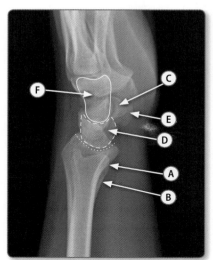

Figure 5.2 Lateral radiograph of the left wrist. (A) Radius (outlined by dotted line), (B) ulna, (C) scaphoid, (D) lunate (outlined by dashed line), (E) pisiform, (F) capitate (outlined by solid line).

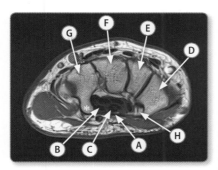

Figure 5.3 Axial T2-weighted magnetic resonance imaging of the left wrist at the level of the carpal tunnel. (A) Flexor retinaculum, (B) tendons of the flexor digitorum profundus and flexor digitorum superficialis in the carpal tunnel, (C) median nerve, (D) trapezium, (E) trapezoid, (F) capitate, (G) hamate, (H) ulnar nerve in the separate ulnar (Guyon's) canal. The hook of hamate (*) is also visible.

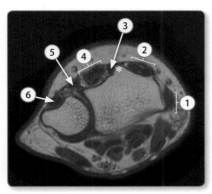

Figure 5.4 Axial T2-weighted MRI of the right wrist, showing the compartments of the extensor tendon. (1) Abductor pollicis longus and extensor pollicis brevis, (2) extensor carpi radialis longus and brevis, (3) extensor pollicis longus, (4) extensor digitorum and extensor indicis, (5) extensor digiti minimi, (6) extensor carpi ulnaris. The radial (Lister's) tubercle (*) is visible.

Compartment	Tendon(s) in compartment
1	Abductor pollicis longus and extensor pollicis brevis
2	Extensor carpi radialis longus and brevis
3	Extensor pollicis longus
4	Extensor digitorum and extensor indicis
5	Extensor digiti minimi
6	Extensor carpi ulnaris

Table 5.1 The extensor tendon compartments of the wrist

5.2 Distal forearm fractures

Fractures of the distal radius and ulna are very common. They usually result from a fall onto an outstretched hand.

Key facts

- Many distal forearm fractures are eponymous (**Table 5.2**).
- Colles fractures are the commonest distal forearm injury, especially in elderly people with osteoporosis (**Figure 5.5**).

Radiological findings

Radiography Fracture lines appear as lucencies traversing the bone in displaced fractures. In impacted fractures, sclerotic lines may be present.

Key imaging findings

- Many forearm fractures involve both the radius and the ulna. It is important to look for secondary injuries such as dislocations or smaller associated fractures.
- The ulnar styloid process is commonly fractured in distal radial fractures.

Eponym	Definition
Colles fracture	Extra-articular fracture with dorsal displacement and angulation (**Figure 5.5**)
Smith fracture	Fracture of the distal radius, with volar displacement and angulation (the opposite of a Colles fracture; **Figure 5.6**)
Barton fracture	Intra-articular fracture of the distal radius (which can be volar or dorsal, depending on its displacement), with dislocation of the radiocarpal joint (**Figure 5.7**)
Galeazzi fracture	Fracture of the distal radial diaphysis and dislocation of the distal radioulnar joint (**Figure 4.6**)
Monteggia fracture	Fracture of the ulnar diaphysis and dislocation of the radial head (elbow dislocation; **Figure 4.7**)

Table 5.2 The many eponymous fractures of the forearm

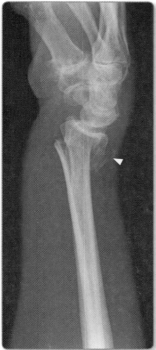

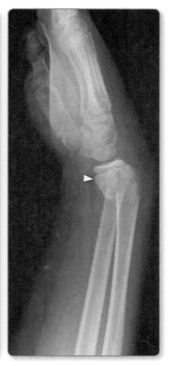

Figure 5.5 Lateral radiograph of the left wrist, showing a comminuted Colles fracture. The distal radial fracture fragment (arrowhead) is displaced dorsally. The surrounding soft tissue is swollen.

Figure 5.6 Lateral radiograph of the left wrist, showing a Smith fracture with volar displacement of the distal radial fracture fragment (arrowhead).

- Because of the plasticity of paediatric bones, fracture patterns in children differ from those in adults (**Table 5.3**).

Treatment

The treatment of distal forearm fractures entirely depends on the degree of displacement, associated injuries and intra-articular involvement. Surgical reduction and internal fixation is reserved

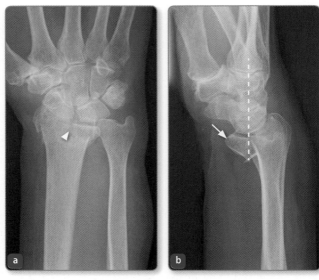

Figure 5.7 (a) Anteroposterior and (b) lateral radiographs of the left wrist, showing a volar-type Barton fracture with volar displacement of the distal radial fragment (arrow). This is an intra-articular extension fracture (arrowhead). The radiocarpal joint is dislocated, and there is loss of alignment between the carpal bones (white line). The distal radius is shown (dashed line).

Eponym	Appearance
Greenstick fracture	This fracture involves a single side of the bone, which becomes convex at the time of injury. On the other side of the bone, cortical integrity is preserved. Thus the fracture resembles damaged green wood, which when bent, breaks on one side only (**Figure 5.8**).
Torus or buckle fracture	Typically visible as small irregularities in the smooth contour of the cortex, which make the surface look bumpy and wrinkled (**Figure 5.9**).
Bowing fracture	No visible fracture line or cortical irregularity, but exaggerated bowing of the diaphysis is seen (**Figure 5.9**).

Table 5.3 Types of forearm fractures in children

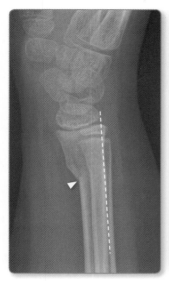

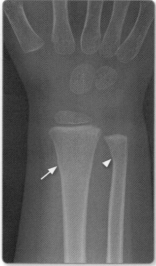

Figure 5.8 Lateral radiograph of the left wrist, showing a greenstick fracture of the volar cortex of the distal radius (arrowhead). The dorsal cortex (outlined in dashed line) remains intact.

Figure 5.9 Anteroposterior radiograph of the left wrist, showing the crinkly appearance of the distal radius (arrow). This finding is consistent with a buckle fracture. The exaggerated angulation of the distal ulna (arrowhead) is consistent with a bowing fracture.

for complex injuries. A conventional cast with immobilisation suffices for less serious injuries.

5.3 Carpal injuries

Scaphoid fractures are the most common carpal fracture. They usually occur after a fall onto an outstretched hand (**Figure 5.10**).

The scaphoid bone is supplied by distal branches of the radial artery. These branches resemble fish hooks going into the distal pole and waist of the bone. A fracture through the waist of the scaphoid bone puts the proximal pole of the scaphoid at risk of avascular osteonecrosis and non-union. Non-union is an important complication of scaphoid injuries.

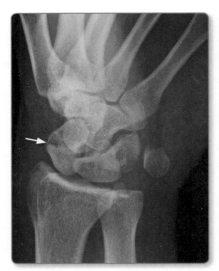

Figure 5.10 Oblique radiograph of the left wrist, showing a fracture of the scaphoid (arrow).

The scaphoid is the carpal bone most likely to fracture. However, hamate and triquetral fractures are also common and have characteristic findings on plain radiograph.

A fall onto the dorsal aspect of an extended wrist is the usual mechanism of injury for wrist dislocations and scapholunate dissociations. These significant soft tissue injuries of the wrist can progress to devastating instability and early degenerative changes.

Key facts

- Because of the intricate ligamentous stabilisation of the carpal bones, scaphoid fractures are often radiographically occult. Magnetic resonance imaging (MRI) is often needed to confirm the diagnosis.
- Disruption of the scapholunate ligament widens the gap between the scaphoid and lunate bones. This widening predisposes the wrist to instability and consequent early osteoarthritis.

Radiological findings

Radiography As in long bones, fractures of the carpal bones are usually identified by cortical breech and displacement of the fracture fragments. The intercarpal joints should all be equidistant. Widening of the gap between any of the carpal bones suggests ligamentous injury.

Computerised tomography This is very useful for evaluating subtle cortical breaks and assessing radiographically occult fragmentation of fractures. However, computerised tomography is not the best modality for assessing soft tissue injuries; it is commonly reserved for preoperative planning for complex carpal injuries.

Magnetic resonance imaging This imaging modality plays a crucial role in confirming the diagnosis of a radiographically occult scaphoid fracture. Fractures are best shown as low-signal lines on coronal T1-weighted acquisitions, with the surrounding fluid signal representing secondary bone marrow oedema (**Figure 5.11**).

Magnetic resonance imaging is also the modality of choice for assessing soft tissue abnormalities in the carpus; it is

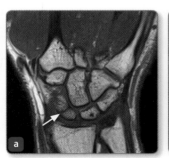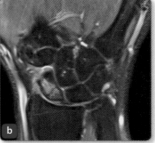

Figure 5.11 (a) T1-weighted and (b) short T1 inversion recovery (STIR) coronal MRI of right wrist, showing a scaphoid waist fracture (arrow; not visible on the corresponding radiograph). Surrounding bone oedema is visible on STIR.

particularly useful for confirming scapholunate ligament tears. Tears are best depicted on T2-weighted sequences, with fluid traversing the ligament fibres.

Key imaging findings

- **Fractures of the hook of hamate** may be very subtle. These fractures result in characteristic indistinct visualisation or non-visualisation of the hook on standard anteroposterior radiographs (**Figure 5.12**).
- **A triquetral fracture** appears on the radiograph as a fleck of bone on the dorsal aspect of the mid carpus, with swelling of the overlying soft tissue (**Figure 5.13**).
- **Widening of the scapholunate interval** is abnormal. A scapholunate interval of > 3 mm is a secondary sign of a scapholunate ligament tear (**Figure 5.14**). This widening is called the Madonna or Terry Thomas sign, because the bones resemble the gap between the upper incisors of these two celebrities.
- **In perilunate dislocations**, the distal radius and the lunate remain aligned on the lateral radiograph. However, the capitate is dorsally dislocated relative to the lunate (**Figure 5.15**).
- **In lunate dislocations**, the lunate is anteriorly dislocated relative to the distal radius. The capitate is not significantly displaced (**Figure 5.16**).

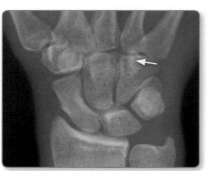

Figure 5.12
Anteroposterior radiograph of the right wrist, showing a poorly visualised hook of hamate (arrow). This indistinct appearance is consistent with a fracture.

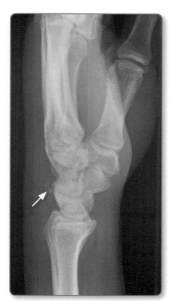

Figure 5.13 Lateral radiograph of the right wrist, showing a fleck of bone (arrow) overlying the mid carpal region. This appearance is consistent with a triquetral fracture.

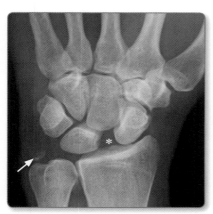

Figure 5.14 Anteroposterior radiograph of the left wrist, showing the so-called Madonna or Terry-Thomas sign of a increased scapholunate interval (> 3 mm, *). A fracture of the ulnar styloid (arrow) is also present.

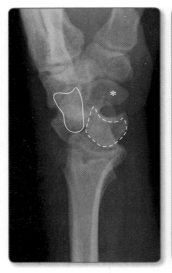

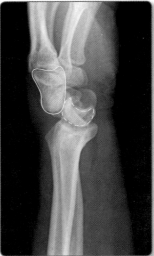

Figure 5.15 Lateral radiograph of the left wrist, showing perilunate dislocation. The lunate (outlined in dashed line) remains aligned with the distal radius. However, the capitate (outlined in solid line) is dislocated dorsally relative to the lunate. There is scapholunate dislocation with a dislocated scaphoid (*).

Figure 5.16 Lateral radiograph of the left wrist, showing lunate dislocation. The lunate (outlined in dashed line) has complete loss of articulation with the distal radius. However, the capitate (outlined in solid line) remains aligned.

Treatment

Arrange a surgical review and further opinion in cases of wrist dislocation or scapholunate tear. Scaphoid fractures are treated with immobilisation and cast. Careful follow-up is needed to monitor for avascular necrosis and non-union.

5.4 Hand injuries

Fractures of the hand can be divided into isolated bony fractures and combination injuries. Isolated bony fractures usually result from a direct impact. Combination injuries occur secondary to hypermobilisation of the joint causing avulsions of tendons or ligaments.

Hand injuries can be classified as shown in **Table 5.4**.

Key facts

- Phalangeal avulsion injuries occur on the dorsal and volar aspect of the bone, depending on the mechanism of injury.
    - Hyperextension occurs in volar plate injuries.
    - Hyperflexion occurs in dorsal plate injuries.

Injury	Description
Bennett fracture	Intra-articular fracture of the base of the metacarpal, with a residual fragment articulating with the trapezium (**Figure 5.17**)
Rolando fracture	A comminuted Bennett fracture (**Figure 5.18**)
Gamekeeper's or skier's thumb	Fracture of the base of the proximal phalanx secondary to disruption of the ulnar collateral ligament (**Figure 5.19**)

Table 5.4 Classification of hand injuries

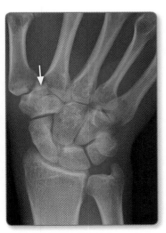

Figure 5.17 Anteroposterior radiograph of the left wrist, showing a Bennett fracture and an intra-articular fracture of the base of the metacarpal. A residual fragment (arrow) is articulating with the trapezium.

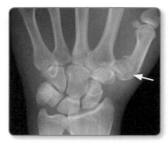

Figure 5.18 Anteroposterior radiograph of the right wrist, showing a Rolando fracture (a comminuted Bennett fracture; arrow).

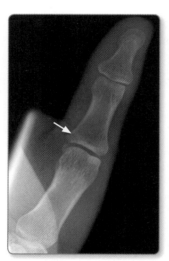

Figure 5.19 Anteroposterior radiograph of the right thumb showing the so-called gamekeeper's or skier's thumb injury: fracture (arrow) of the base of the proximal phalanx secondary to disruption of the ulnar collateral ligament.

Radiological findings

Radiography Radiographically, phalangeal avulsion injuries usually show a small fleck of bone near the joint on the volar or dorsal aspect of the affected bone. Stress views may accentuate the fracture line in avulsion injuries.

Isolated metacarpal and phalangeal fractures have similar fracture characteristics to those of long bones.

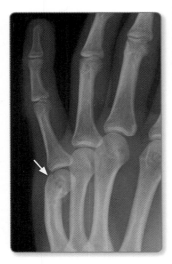

Figure 5.20 Anteroposterior radiograph of the left hand, showing the so-called boxer's fracture (arrow), which is a fracture of the metacarpal neck caused by punching something (or someone).

Key imaging findings

- A fracture of the metacarpal neck caused by punching something (or someone) is called a boxer's fracture. Boxer's fractures are most commonly seen in the 5th metacarpal, with volar displacement of the distal fracture fragment (**Figure 5.20**).
- Localised soft tissue swelling around a joint may provide a clue to the site of injury.

Treatment

Bennett and Rolando fractures may need open reduction to preserve the vital function of the thumb. Simple hand fractures can commonly be treated conservatively by immobilising the injured digit by strapping it to its neighbours.

5.5 De Quervain's disease

De Quervain's disease is a tendinopathy and stenosing tenosynovitis of the abductor pollicis longus and extensor pollicis brevis tendons of the 1st extensor compartment of the wrist joint.

Key facts

- De Quervain's disease is commonest in middle-aged women. The disease is bilateral in ≤ 30% of patients.
- Patients complain of pain and swelling at or along the radial styloid region.
- De Quervain's disease is typically idiopathic but may present after acute or repetitive trauma.
- The disease is associated with systemic conditions such as rheumatoid arthritis, gout and hypothyroidism.

Radiological findings

Ultrasound A longitudinal ultrasound scan shows diffuse distension of the tendon sheath, with surrounding fluid hypoechogenicity. A transverse scan shows a double-target pattern. Affected tendons may be thickened but sometimes appear normal.

Magnetic resonance imaging There is a fluid signal in the common tendon sheath of the abductor pollicis longus and the extensor pollicis brevis, with surrounding soft tissue oedema. Tendon thickening, signal changes or both may be present in severe cases.

Key imaging findings

- There is a typical tenosynovitis appearance in the 1st extensor tendon compartment (**Figure 5.21**).
- The abductor pollicis longus or extensor pollicis brevis tendons may be hypertrophied or normal (**Figure 5.22**).

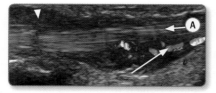

Figure 5.21 Longitudinal ultrasound showing tendinopathic abductor pollicis longus (A). There is a grossly increased amount of fluid (arrowhead) in the tendon sheath, which also shows increased Doppler flow (long arrow). These findings are consistent with tenosynovitis.

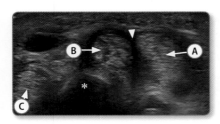

Figure 5.22 Transverse ultrasound showing hypertrophied abductor pollicis longus Ⓐ and heterogeneous extensor pollicis brevis Ⓑ. There is increased fluid in the tendon sheath (arrowhead) in the 1st extensor tendon compartment of the distal radius (*). The extensor carpi radialis longus Ⓒ in the adjacent 2nd compartment is normal.

Treatment

As with most cases of tendinosis, de Quervain's disease may be self-limiting. Splints and anti-inflammatory medication are the first-line treatment. Corticosteroid injection can improve symptoms in prolonged cases. Surgical release of the compartment may be needed if conservative treatment fails.

5.6 Triangular fibrocartilage complex pathology

The triangular fibrocartilage complex can be injured by acute trauma (class 1 injuries) or degenerative changes (class 2 injuries). Class 1 (traumatic) injuries are usually caused by a fall onto an extended wrist with the forearm in pronation, or by a traction injury to the ulnar side of the wrist. Class 2 (degenerative) injuries are associated with positive ulnar variance, ulnocarpal impaction or both.

Key facts

- The triangular fibrocartilage complex comprises a central articular disc, meniscus homologue and extensor carpi ulnaris subsheath, as well as radioulnar and ulnocarpal ligaments.
- Patients present with wrist pain on the side of the ulna, frequently with clicking.

Radiological findings

Radiography Radiographic findings are usually normal, but ulnar variance can be assessed on a posteroanterior view.

Magnetic resonance imaging Tears of the triangular fibrocartilage complex can be seen on MRI. However, sensitivity is much improved with an MRI wrist arthrogram, which has replaced the traditional arthrogram.

Key imaging findings
- **Class 1** traumatic injuries are classified as a central perforation (A) or avulsion at the ulnar (B), distal (C) or radial (D) aspects, which can have associated fractures.
- **Class 2** degenerative injuries are classified in a range from A to E, depending on wear or perforation and the presence of ulnocarpal chondromalacia or arthropathy.
- Pooling of contrast in the distal radioulnar joint is a feature of **class 1A** central perforations (**Figure 5.23**). Contrast pooling is visible on the initial arthrogram (**Figure 5.24**).

Treatment
Many injuries to the triangular fibrocartilage complex can be treated conservatively. Arthroscopic debridement or repair

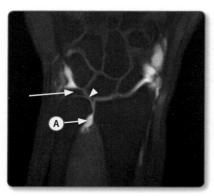

Figure 5.23 Coronal T1-weighted magnetic resonance imaging of the right wrist with fat saturation, showing contrast pooling in the distal radial ulnar joint (**A**). Pooling occurs because of a central perforation (arrowhead) of the triangular fibrocartilage complex (long arrow).

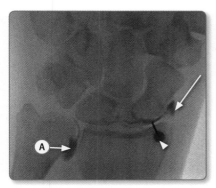

Figure 5.24
Anteroposterior
arthrogram of the right
wrist, showing needle
(arrowhead) with contrast
in the joint space (long
arrow). The contrast tracks
into the distal radioulnar
joint space (A).

is done for persistently symptomatic cases. Various surgical procedures can be used to correct ulnar variance.

5.7 Ulnar collateral ligament of thumb injuries

This ligament is on the ulnar side of the metacarpophalangeal joint of the thumb. It can be injured by an acute valgus force (in skier's thumb) or by chronic repetitive strain (in game-keeper's thumb). A full-thickness tear results in instability of the metacarpophalangeal joint of the thumb, causing pain.

Key facts

- Stress radiographs are no longer done. They are inaccurate and may worsen the condition.
- The spectrum of injuries to the ulnar collateral ligament includes strain and partial- or full-thickness tears.
- Associated avulsion fracture of the base of the metacarpal may be present.

Radiological findings

Radiograph An associated avulsion fracture of the ulnar side of the base of the proximal phalanx may be visible (**Figure 5.25**).

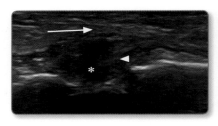

Figure 5.25 Longitudinal ultrasound view of the thumb, showing the metacarpophalangeal joint on the ulnar side. There is a full-thickness tear in the ulnar collateral ligament (arrowhead), which contains the associated fluid (*). The overlying adductor aponeurosis (arrow) remains intact, and no Stener lesion is present.

Ultrasound This is the modality of choice, because dynamic imaging can assess this superficial ligament very well. Ultrasound is used to assess the degree of tear and to identify any associated displacement.

A full-thickness ulnar collateral ligament tear with proximal retraction causing the ligament to lie superficial to the adductor aponeurosis creates an irregular, lobulated nodule. This nodule is diagnostic of a Stener lesion.

Magnetic resonance imaging This is usually unnecessary if ultrasound expertise is available. The typical low-signal appearance of the ligament on MRI can show a tear with retraction. It can also clarify whether the adductor aponeurosis blocks the apposition of torn ends.

Key imaging findings
- Assess the sprain and extent of tear in the ulnar collateral ligament.
  - Ligament sprain is visible as thickening.
  - Tears can be partial thickness (in an incomplete defect) or full thickness (in a complete defect).
- A Stener lesion appears as nodular thickening superficial to the adductor aponeurosis. The nodule resemble a yo-yo.
- Use dynamic movements of the interphalangeal joint of the thumb to check the sliding of the adductor aponeurosis over the ulnar collateral ligament. The aponeurosis slides smoothly over the ligament if there is no Stener lesion.

Treatment

Surgical repair is needed in cases of acute presentation of a full-thickness tear. Partial-thickness tears can be treated conservatively, for example by using a thumb spica for 6 weeks. A Stener lesion hinders ligament healing and is an indication for surgical repair, because conservative management may result in permanent instability of the metacarpophalangeal joint.

Pelvic girdle and hip

6.1 Key anatomy

The pelvic girdle is formed from five bones: the ilium, the ischium, the pubis, the sacrum and the coccyx (**Figure 6.1**). The ilium, ischium and pubis fuse to form the acetabulum, a socket for the femoral head at the hip joint.

Whereas the head of the humerus lies in the shallow glenoid fossa of the shsoulder joint, the head of the femur sits deep in the acetabulum of the hip joint. This arrangement of femoral head and acetabulum provides more stability but allows a smaller range of movement.

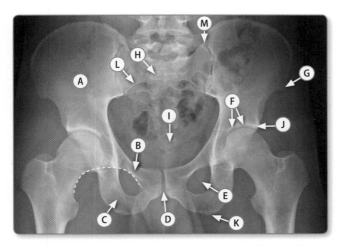

Figure 6.1 Anteroposterior radiograph of the pelvis and hips. (A) Illium, (B) pubis, (C) ischium, (D) pubic symphysis, (E) obturator foramen, (F) acetabulum, (G) anterior superior iliac spine, (H) sacrum, (I) coccyx, (J) anterior inferior iliac spine, (K) ischial tuberosity, (L) arcuate line of sacrum, (M) sacroiliac joint. Shenton's line (dashed line) follows the inferior margin of the femoral neck and head and continues along the superior pubic ramus.

The acetabular labrum is a ring of cartilage around the acetabulum. The labrum helps stabilise the hip joint by deepening the socket.

Figures 6.2 and **6.3** show the appearance of the pelvis on magnetic resonance imaging (MRI).

Imaging points
- When imaging the hip in trauma, obtain a cross-table projection (**Figure 6.4**) as well as an anteroposterior view of the pelvic (**Figure 6.5**)
- The pelvis can be considered a ring of bone. A fracture in one part of the ring usually indicates a fracture on another part of it
- Shenton's line follows the inferior margin of the femoral neck and head and continues along the superior pubic ramus

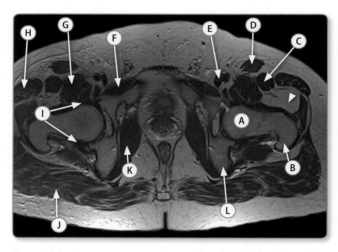

Figure 6.2 Axial magnetic resonance imaging of the pelvis at the level of the hip joints. (A) Femoral head, (B) greater trochanter, (C) rectus femoris (incidental lipoma posteriorly, arrowhead), (D) sartorius, (E) common femoral vessels, (F) pectineus, (G) iliopsoas, (H) tensor fascia latae, (I) anterior and posterior acetabular labrum, (J) gluteus maximus, (K) obturator internus, (L) ischium.

(**Figure 6.1**). If Shenton's line is disrupted in a pelvic radiograph from an adult, a fracture of the femoral neck or pubic rami should be suspected

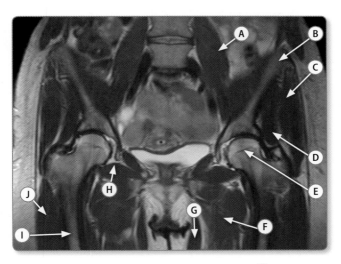

Figure 6.3 Coronal magnetic resonance imaging of the pelvis. (A) Psoas major, (B) ilium, (C) gluteus maximus, (D) gluteus medius, (E) femoral head, (F) adductor magnus, (G) gracilis, (H) obturator externus, (I) femoral shaft, (J) vastus lateralis.

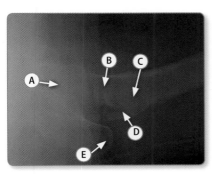

Figure 6.4 Cross-table lateral radiograph of the right hip. (A) Femoral head, (B) femoral neck, (C) lesser trochanter, (D) greater trochanter, (E) ischial tuberosity.

- Hilgenreiner's line is a horizontal line drawn between the superior aspect of both triradiate cartilages in a pelvic radiograph from a child. Perkin's line is a vertical line perpendicular to Hilgenreiner's line. Perkin's line intersects the most lateral part of the acetabular roof. The upper femoral epiphysis should lie in the inferomedial quadrant formed by these lines (**Figure 6.6**).

Clinical insight

Be sure to request the correct radiographic view. A pelvic radiograph will show the entire pelvis, whereas a bilateral hip radiograph will show both hip joints and the proximal femora and not the superior portion of the pelvis including the iliac crest.

6.2 Avulsion fractures of the pelvis

Acute avulsion injuries of the pelvis occur in adolescents as a result of sudden muscle contraction at the point of attachment to the growth plate. Patients present with localised pain and weakness. Common locations for pelvic avulsion fractures are listed in **Table 6.1**.

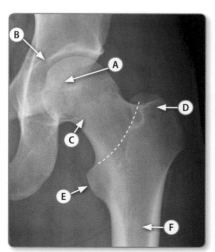

Figure 6.5 Anteroposterior radiograph of the left hip. Ⓐ Femoral head, Ⓑ acetabulum, Ⓒ femoral neck, Ⓓ greater trochanter, Ⓔ lesser trochanter, Ⓕ proximal femoral shaft. The intertrochanteric line (dashed line) is shown.

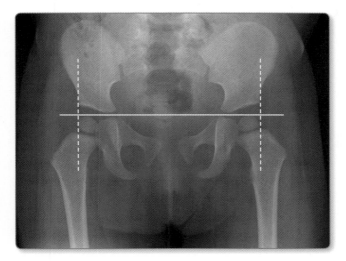

Figure 6.6 Anteroposterior radiograph of a child's pelvis. The horizontal white line is Hilgenreiner's line. The vertical lines are Perkin's. The upper femoral epiphysis normally lies in the inferomedial quadrant formed by these lines.

Key facts

- The correct diagnosis is based on the history and the radiographic location of the avulsed bony fragment.
- Chronic injuries may occur with repetitive stress.
- The ischial tuberosity is the most common site of injury, followed by the iliac spines.

Radiological findings

Radiography The bony fragments are curvilinear and are located close to the muscle origin. Subacute and chronic injuries can appear aggressive and may therefore be confused with tumours and infections. Bone forms between the fragment and the apophysis during healing.

Computerised tomography For acute injuries, computerised tomography (CT) is unnecessary. However, it can be useful for delayed presentation or chronic injuries.

Bony origin	Muscle(s)	Apophysis appearance (years of age)	Apophysis closure (years of age)	Typical history
Anterior superior iliac spine (**Figure 6.7**)	Sartorius	13–15	21–25	Running
Anterior inferior iliac spine (**Figure 6.8**)	Rectus femoris	13–14	16–18	Sprinting or soccer
Ischial tuberosity (**Figure 6.9**)	Hamstrings	14–16	18–21	Hurdling
Iliac crest	Abdominal wall muscles	12–15	18–21	Indirect trauma
Inferior pubic ramus	Adductor muscles	–	–	Gymnastics
Greater trochanter	External rotator muscles	4	16–18	Running
Lesser trochanter	Iliopsoas	8–12	16–18	Kicking sports

Table 6.1 Bony sites and muscles involved in various avulsion injuries

Magnetic resonance imaging Fluid-sensitive fat-suppressed sequences show bone marrow oedema at the origin site (**Figure 6.10**).

Key imaging finding

- A bony fragment avulsed from an appropriate anatomical muscle origin is visible (see **Table 6.1**).

Treatment

Treatment is conservative: bed rest, pain relief and protected weight bearing followed by physiotherapy. Large displaced bony fragments are treated with open reduction and fixation.

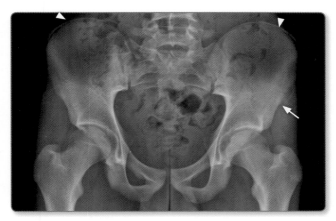

Figure 6.7 Anteroposterior radiograph of the pelvis, showing avulsion of the left anterior superior iliac spine (arrrow) caused by an avulsion injury of the sartorius. Note the normal unfused iliac crest apophysis bilaterally (arrowheads).

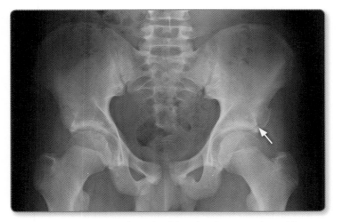

Figure 6.8 Anteroposterior radiograph of the pelvis, showing avulsion of the left anterior inferior iliac spine (arrow) caused by an avulsion injury of the rectus femoris.

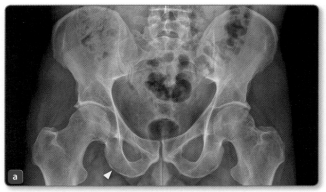

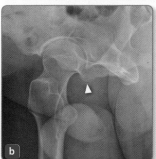

Figure 6.9 (a) Anteroposterior radiograph of the pelvis, showing a subtle fracture line (arrowhead) at the right ischial tuberosity. (b) A right oblique radiograph confirms an ischial tuberosity avulsion fracture (arrowhead).

6.3 Pelvic fractures

The pelvis comprises one large bony ring and two smaller bony rings. The large bony ring is formed by the iliac wings joined to the sacrum. The smaller bony rings are formed by the pubic and ischial bones joined at the pubic symphysis.

The anteroposterior view is standard. Judet (45° oblique) views can also be obtained to assess the anterior and posterior columns.

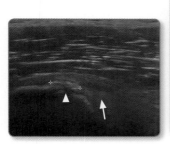 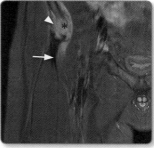

Figure 6.10 (a) Longitudinal ultrasound of the anterior right inferior iliac spine and (b) coronal T2-weighted magnetic resonance imaging (MRI), showing a fracture (arrowhead) with avulsion of the cortical fragment (between the + signs). The cortical fragment is attached to the origin of the rectus femoris tendon (arrow). Surrounding haematoma and soft tissue changes (*) are visible on MRI.

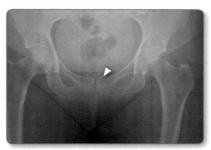

Figure 6.11
Anteroposterior radiograph of the hip, showing a fracture of the left superior pubic ramus (arrowhead).

Key facts

- Pelvic fractures can be stable or unstable.
  - Stable fractures are single breaks in the bony ring. They are caused by moderate trauma. Fractures of a single pubic ramus (**Figure 6.11**), the iliac wing (Duverney fractures), and the sacrum or coccyx, as well as avulsion fractures, are stable.
  - Unstable fractures are caused by double breaks in the bony ring. They are caused by severe trauma, such as

that sustained in road traffic collisions. **Straddle** fractures (involving all four pubic rami), **Malgaigne** fractures (vertical shears; **Figure 6.12**), dislocations and open-book fractures (**Figure 6.13**) are unstable.

- In children, the synchondrosis between the ischial and pubic bones can simulate healing fractures.
- The sacroiliac joint widths should be equal.
- In the symphysis pubis, the superior surfaces of the pubic rami should align, with a joint width of ≤ 5 mm in adolescents and ≤ 10 mm in adults.
- Widening of both the symphysis pubis and the sacroiliac joint indicates an unstable fracture.

Radiological findings

Assess the radiological lines (see section 6.1, *Key anatomy*).

- Fractures show loss of cortical continuity or sclerotic lines with overlapping bone fragments.
- Sacroiliac joints may be ≤ 4 mm in adults.
- Widening of the symphysis pubis indicates disruption.
- In the sacral foramina, disruption of the curved arcuate line indicates fracture.
- Compare the acetabulum (**Figure 6.14**) with that on other side and use Judet views.

Radiography All patients with pelvic trauma should undergo radiography. A cross-table lateral view can be used in selected

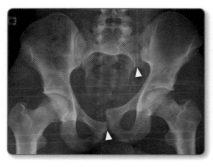

Figure 6.12
Anteroposterior radiograph of the pelvis, showing a Malgaigne (vertical shear) fracture. This type of fracture is unstable. There is vertical disruption of the symphysis pubis and left sacroiliac joint, with associated fractures and likely underlying ligamentous injuries (arrowheads).

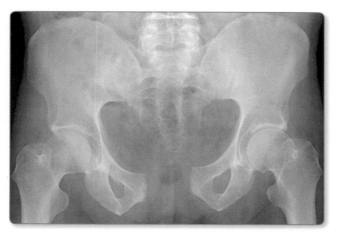

Figure 6.13 Anteroposterior radiograph of the pelvis, showing an open book type of fracture resulting from an anteroposterior compression injury. The injury disrupts the symphysis pubis so that the pelvis opens like a book. Disruption of the sacroiliac joint is usually present but may not be visible on radiograph.

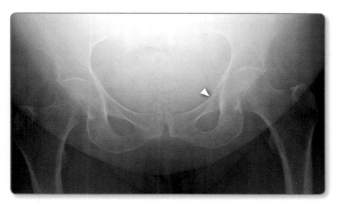

Figure 6.14 Anteroposterior radiograph of the hip, showing a left acetabular fracture (arrowhead).

cases. Judet views, i.e. side views of the pelvis rotated 45° anteriorly, are helpful to assess acetabular fractures.

Ultrasound This is used to identify associated pelvic and abdominal soft tissue trauma.

Computerised tomography This is useful for identifying sacral fractures and loose bodies after dislocation. CT can also be used to assess the acetabulum. However, CT findings rarely change management compared with good plain films including Judet views.

Magnetic resonance imaging Although not indicated for acute pelvic trauma, MRI is useful for assessing soft tissues.

Key imaging findings
- Cortical breaks and loss of continuity
- Disruption of normal alignment

Treatment
Compression and shear fractures can cause life-threatening haemorrhage. Unstable fractures need fixation.

6.4 Femoral neck fractures

Fractures of the femoral neck are common in the elderly and can be subtle. A history of injury may not always be present. The patient may have a shortened externally rotated leg if the fracture is displaced.

Key facts
- Initial radiographs can be normal but repeat imaging is indicated for persisting symptoms.
- Essential views are an anteroposterior view of the whole pelvis (**Figure 6.15**) and hip joints and a lateral view of the painful hip.
- Femoral neck fractures can be intracapsular or extracapsular.
  - Subcapital, midcervical and basicervical fractures are intracapsular. Intracapsular fractures are at increased risk of avascular necrosis and non-union. Subcapital

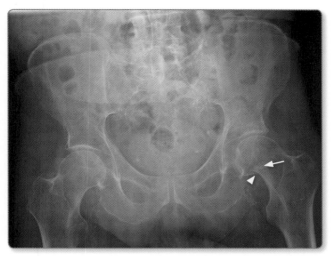

Figure 6.15 Anteroposterior radiograph of the pelvis, showing a sclerotic band (arrow) at the right neck of femur, proven to be an impacted fracture. Note disruption of Shenton's line (arrowhead).

fractures are common, midcervical fractures are rare and basicervical fractures are uncommon.
- Intertrochanteric (**Figure 6.16**) and subtrochanteric fractures are extracapsular.

Radiological findings

Radiography Look for a break or step in the cortical contours of the femoral neck. Discontinuity of trabecular pattern and loss of Shenton's line also indicate a fracture. CT and MRI are useful when the diagnosis is uncertain.

Computerised tomography This is indicated for suspected femoral neck fractures with normal radiographs, as well as posterior hip dislocation. CT is used to look for associated acetabular injury and loose bodies. CT is faster than MRI and less prone to motion artefact.

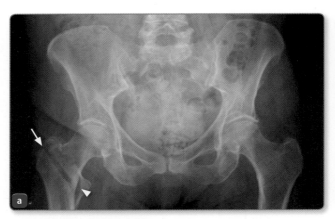

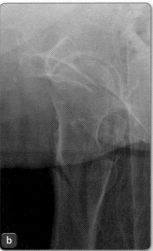

Figure 6.16 (a) Anteroposterior and (b) lateral radiographs of the pelvis, showing a right intertrochanteric fracture of the right proximal femur. The fracture extends into the greater trochanter (arrow) and the lesser trochanter (arrowhead).

Magnetic resonance imaging Limited MRIs with T1-weighted and short T1 inversion recovery (STIR) coronal sequences show femoral neck fractures and soft tissues injuries.

Key imaging findings
- Shenton's line is lost in displaced fractures.
- Impacted fractures may appear as a sclerotic line.

Treatment
Intracapsular fractures usually need femoral head replacement with hemiarthroplasty or total hip replacement. Extracapsular fractures can be treated with reduction and internal fixation, often with a dynamic hip screw.

6.5 Developmental dysplasia of the hip

About 1% of newborns have developmental dysplasia of the hip. The condition was previously called congenital dislocation of the hip. However, the condition is not always congenital, and not all cases involve dislocation.

Key facts
- Pathological findings range from mild acetabular dysplasia to frankly dislocated hip with dysmorphic femoral head and acetabulum.
- Screening involves routine examination of all newborns. Imaging is done if developmental dysplasia of the hip is suspected or if the newborn is at high risk for the condition (breech birth increases risk).

Radiological findings

Radiography Anteroposterior views of the pelvis show symmetric ossification centres of the femoral epiphyses.

Ultrasound In children younger than 6 months, ultrasound is used to assess hip shape and stability. Ultrasound in the coronal plane is used to measure acetabular concavity (the α angle) and cartilaginous roof coverage (the β angle), as well as acetabular maturity (*d/D*).

Computerised tomography This is useful for evaluation of complicated dislocations as well as for postoperative evaluation of the hip.

Magnetic resonance imaging Scans can be used to detect complications of developmental dysplasia of the hip and its treatment, such as avascular necrosis.

Key imaging findings
- On anteroposterior radiographs, both femoral heads should be in the inner inferior quadrants formed by the intersection of Hilgenreiner's and Perkin's lines (see **Figure 6.6**). Shenton's line should be continuous.
- In ultrasound scans in the coronal plane, the α angle should be > 60° and the β angle should be < 55° (see **Figure 6.17**).

Treatment
Hip instability can be treated with a hip spica or harness if the baby is < 6 months old. If developmental dysplasia of the hip is diagnosed in a child aged > 6 months, or if non-operative management has failed, closed reduction may be necessary. Open reduction (and acetabular surgery) is done for children aged > 2 years.

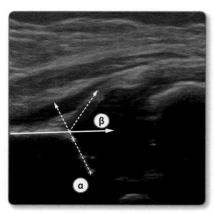

Figure 6.17 Longitudinal ultrasound scan in the coronal plane, showing the alpha angle (α) between the baseline (solid arrow), and the roof line (dashed arrow), as well as the beta angle (β) between the baseline and the inclination line (dotted arrow).

6.6 Acetabular labral pathology

The acetabular labrum can be torn by degeneration or trauma. Labral tears present with hip or groin pain and occasionally with clicking or giving way.

Key facts

- Labral tears can be classified by cause, site or shape.
- Femoroacetabular impingement is thought to contribute to degenerative labral tears in younger patients.
  - The cam-type femoroacetabular impingement involves an aspherical femoral head–neck relation resulting from an osseous bump causing a pistol grip deformity (**Figure 6.18**).

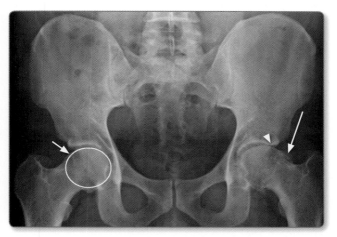

Figure 6.18 Anteroposterior radiograph of the pelvis, showing a minor osseous bump on the right head–neck junction (short arrow) relative to the circle. The large osseous bump on the opposite side (long arrow) caused a pistol grip deformity, consistent with a cam-type femoroacetabular impingement. Note the resulting osteoarthropathy (arrowhead).

- The pincer-type femoroacetabular impingement involves over-coverage of the acetabulum (**Figure 6.19**).
- In mixed-type femoroacetabular impingement, both conditions (cam and pincer) coexist.
- Developmental dysplasia of the hip can contribute to degenerative tears.
- Most labral tears are anterior but they can also be posterior or superolateral. Posterior labral tears are commoner in Japan.
- The commonest shapes are radial flap or radial fibrillated tears. Other types include longitudinal peripheral tears and unstable tears. Unstable tears often cause mechanical symptoms.

Radiological findings

Radiography Anteroposterior pelvic and cross-table lateral views may show developmental dysplasia of the hip or femoroacetabular impingement.

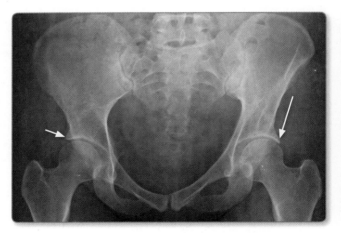

Figure 6.19 Anteroposterior radiograph of the pelvis, showing a normal acetabulum on one side (short arrow) but over-coverage of the acetabulum on the opposite side (long arrow). These findings are consistent with a unilateral pincer-type femoroacetabular impingement.

Magnetic resonance imaging This modality can be used to rule out differential causes of hip and groin pain. However, an MRI arthrogram of the hip is needed to evaluate the labrum (**Figure 6.20**).

Key imaging findings

- To help assess subtle cam-type femoroacetabular impingement, draw a circle to fill the femoral head. Any bony protrusion beyond this circle suggests a cam lesion (**Figure 6.18**).
- The α angle can be measured on radiograph or MRI as the angle between a line drawn from the long axis of the femoral neck and a line drawn from the centre of the femoral head to the head–neck junction. An α angle > 55° indicates a cam lesion.
- Do not mistake a normal sublabral recess for a tear. Normal sublabral recesses do not extend through the full thickness of the labral base. Paralabral cysts can increase the diagnostic certainty of a tear (**Figure 6.21**).

Treatment

If conservative measures fail to control symptoms, or if functional limitations remain unsatisfactory, surgical review by a hip joint specialist is appropriate.

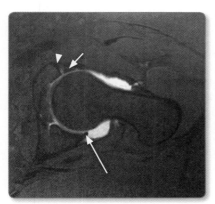

Figure 6.20 Axial T1-weighted magnetic resonance imaging arthrogram of the left hip with fat saturation, showing the tracking of contrast (arrowhead) beneath the anterior labrum (short arrow). This finding is consistent with a full-thickness tear. The posterior labrum (long arrow) is normal.

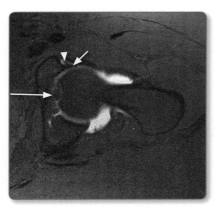

Figure 6.21 Axial T1-weighted magnetic resonance imaging arthrogram of the left hip with fat saturation, showing a paralabral cyst (arrowhead). Paralabral cysts are highly suggestive of an underlying labral tear, even in the absence of contrast tracking beneath the anterior labrum (short arrow). The ligamentum teres (long arrow) is normal.

Hip arthroscopy is the gold standard. It can be used to detect and to repair, debride or excise some tears.

6.7 Slipped upper femoral epiphyses

Slipped upper femoral epiphysis is the commonest adolescent hip pathology. Mechanical and constitutional factors are thought to contribute to slippage of the capital (head) portion of the femur on the physis. The slip can be acute, acute on chronic or chronic. Risk factors include obesity, endocrine disease and delayed puberty.

Key facts

- A slipped upper femoral epiphysis occurs most commonly in boys aged 10–17 years (average age, 12 years).
- Slippage of the contralateral femoral epiphysis occurs in a third of patients, usually in ≤ 6 months.
- Diagnosis is often delayed, especially if the patient presents with only referred knee pain.

Radiological findings

Radiography   Anteroposterior pelvic (**Figure 6.22**) and lateral frog-leg radiographs are essential for diagnosis. Include the contralateral side for comparison. Look for the appearance

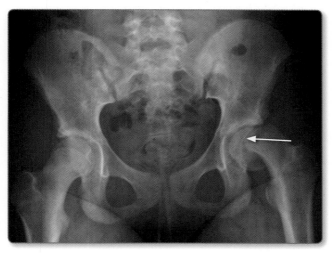

Figure 6.22 Anteroposterior radiograph of the pelvis, showing late presentation of a displaced femoral epiphysis on the left side (arrow).

of melting ice cream (the capital portion of the femur) falling medially onto a cone (the rest of the femoral head and neck). Lateral frog-leg views are the first to show slippage.

Computerised tomography This is a highly sensitive method for detecting early disease. However, because of the radiation involved, CT is reserved for measuring the degree of tilt.

Magnetic resonance imaging Early slippage and marrow oedema can be seen. MRI also helps in follow-up examinations to detect contralateral disease.

Key imaging findings
- Klein's line is a line drawn along the superior border of the proximal femur metaphysis. The line should intersect part of the proximal femoral epiphysis (**Figure 6.23**).
- Increased opacity of the metaphysis or subtle changes associated with early slight widening of the physis may be the only sign of early disease.

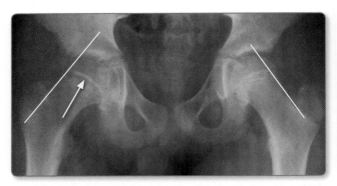

Figure 6.23 Anteroposterior radiograph of the pelvis, showing Klein's line (white) failing to intersect with the right proximal femoral epiphysis on the right hip. There is also widening of the physis and adjacent metaphyseal sclerosis (arrow).

- There is increased signal on T2-weighted MRI, representing marrow oedema from early slippage.

Treatment

The capital head must be stabilised with external in situ (i.e. without attempting reduction) pinning or open reduction and pinning. Delayed treatment can lead to avascular necrosis, chronic pain or long-term degenerative hip disease.

6.8 Perthes disease (Legg–Calvé–Perthes disease)

Perthes disease is an idiopathic osteonecrosis of the femoral head in children. The disease is self-limiting but a resulting deformed femoral head can lead to osteoarthritis in adulthood.

Key facts

- Perthes disease usually affects children aged 4–8 years. Boys are affected 3–5 times more often than girls.
- The disease is bilateral in ≤ 20% of cases, typically in a successive rather than a simultaneous pattern.

- Pathological changes occur in four stages: devascularisation, collapse with fragmentation, reossification and remodelling.

Radiological findings

Radiography Look for a sclerotic femoral head with collapse and sequestration (**Figure 6.24**). Later, the femoral head appears flattened and fragmented. The hip joint space may be widened by cartilage hypertrophy, hip effusion or both.

Computerised tomography First, subtle changes in the trabecular pattern are visible. Later, curvilinear zones of sclerosis and collapse appear. Subchondral fractures with intraosseous cysts are signs of late disease.

Magnetic resonance imaging This is more sensitive for early disease, with irregular foci or linear segments replacing normal signal intensity. The commonest feature is reduced signal

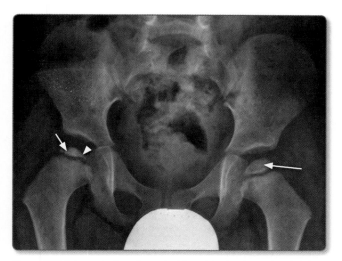

Figure 6.24 Anteroposterior radiograph of the pelvis, showing a sclerotic right femoral epiphysis (short arrow) with minor fragmentation in the medial portion (arrowhead). The left epiphysis (long arrow) is normal in this case.

intensity on T1-weighted MRI and increased signal intensity on STIR, with enhancement indicating viable bone. There is signal void on all sequences, indicating sclerotic dead bone. End-stage healed bone has normal signal intensity.

Key imaging findings

- The appearance of Perthes disease varies greatly, depending on the stage of the disease.
- Magnetic resonance imaging is better for detecting early disease. Look for low T1 and high STIR signal intensity.
- Contrast enhancement on MRI is used to identify viable normal bone.

Treatment

The primary goal is to help recover or preserve the femoral head. Many cases of Perthes disease need only careful watching. The aim of surgery is to obtain adequate containment of the femoral head.

6.9 Avascular necrosis of the hip

The key feature of avascular necrosis of the hip is an ischaemic insult producing interruption of the blood supply to the affected portion of the bone. The duration of interruption depends on the cause.

Table 6.2 shows clinical findings at the five stages of avascular necrosis of the hip.

Stage	Description
0	Clinical suspicion, normal radiographs
1	Clinical findings, abnormal nuclear medicine studies
2	Osteopenia, cysts, bony sclerosis (Figure 6.25)
3	Crescent sign
4	Flattening of femoral head
5	Joint narrowing and acetabular changes

Table 6.2 Clinical findings at the five stages of avascular necrosis of the hip

Key fact

- The typical patient is aged 20–50 years and presents with hip, groin or knee pain. The pain is usually chronic, and the patient has a reduced range of motion.

Radiological findings

Radiography Osteopaenia is a feature of subsequent ischaemia and reactive hyperaemia. Many months may pass before osteopenia is seen on radiograph. Fragmentation is followed by sclerosis (**Figure 6.25**) then demineralisation cysts. The crescent sign is a late feature.

Bone scan A triple-phase bone scan shows reduced uptake in the blood pool phase. Scans from later stages of avascular necrosis show increased uptake, which is consistent with osteoblastic remodelling.

Magnetic resonance imaging For early disease, MRI is the most sensitive imaging modality. Scans show an Irregular,

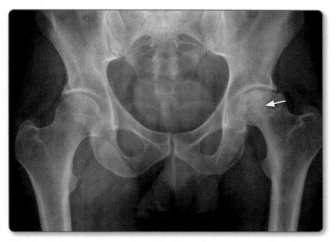

Figure 6.25 Anteroposterior radiograph of the pelvis, showing a collapsed femoral head with sclerosis (arrow), consistent with the late appearance of avascular necrosis.

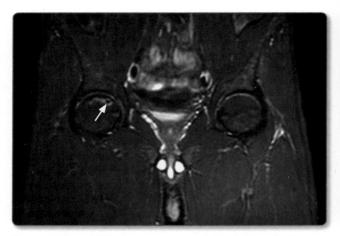

Figure 6.26 Coronal STIR magnetic resonance imaging, showing a focal low signal area with adjacent high-signal oedema of subchondral bone marrow of the left femoral head (arrowhead), consistent with early avascular necrosis.

subchondral, low linear signal in the epiphysis and extending to the subchondral bone (**Figure 6.26**).

Key imaging findings
- There is fragmentation of the epiphysis.
- Variable sclerosis of the femoral head is visible as reossification occurs.
- Demineralisation cysts in the lateral metaphysis are present in some cases.
- Look for the crescent sign: a subchondral fracture, typically on the anterosuperior aspect of the femoral head.
- Also look for the doughnut sign: a persistent central cold spot in a zone of increased uptake.
- The double-line sign is an inner hyperintense line (acute granulation tissue) and an outer hypointense line (sclerosis and fibrosis).

Treatment

Non–weight bearing is the initial conservative management. Core decompression or osteotomy is a surgical option for resistant cases. Long-term degenerative joint disease may need hip arthroplasty.

7.1 Key anatomy

The knee is a hinge joint formed by the articulations of the femur, tibia and patella. The tibiofemoral joint is formed by the articulation between the medial and lateral femoral condyles and the corresponding tibial condyles. The patellofemoral joint is formed by the articulation of the patella and the patella groove of the distal femur. The tibiofemoral joint is partly lined on either side by cartilaginous articular discs called the medial and lateral menisci.

The medial and lateral collateral ligaments support the knee joint on either side. The anterior and posterior cruciate ligaments form an X between the femur and the tibia in the knee joint, with the anterior cruciate ligament inserting lateral to the posterior cruciate ligament.

Figures 7.1 and **7.2** show the appearance of the knee on radiograph. **Figures 7.3–7.5** show the knee on magnetic resonance imaging.

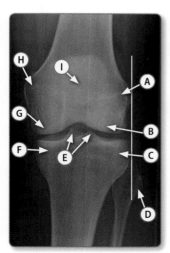

Figure 7.1 Anteroposterior radiograph of the left knee. No more than 5 mm of tibial condyle should be visible lateral to a vertical line drawn at the lateral femoral condyle (line). (A) Lateral femoral epicondyle, (B) lateral femoral condyle, (C) lateral tibial plateau, (D) fibular head, (E) tibial spines, (F) medial tibial plateau, (G) medial femoral condyle, (H) medial femoral epicondyle, (I) patella.

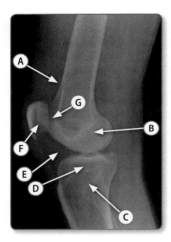

Figure 7.2 Lateral radiograph of the left knee. (A) Suprapatellar fat pad, (B) femoral condyles, (C) fibular head, (D) tibial plateau, (E) infrapatellar fat pad, (F) patella, (G) patellofemoral joint.

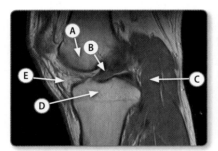

Figure 7.3 Sagittal T1-weighted magnetic resonance imaging of the left knee at the level of the anterior cruciate ligament. (A) Femoral condyle, (B) anterior cruciate ligament, (C) lateral head of gastrocnemius, (D) tibial plateau, (E) infrapatellar fat pad.

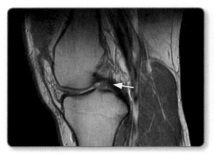

Figure 7.4 Sagittal T1-weighted magnetic resonance imaging of the left knee at the level of the posterior cruciate ligament (arrow).

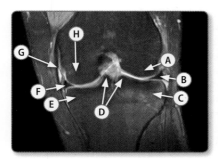

Figure 7.5 Coronal STIR magnetic resonance imaging of the left knee. Ⓐ Lateral femoral condyle, Ⓑ lateral meniscus, Ⓒ lateral tibial plateau, Ⓓ tibial spines, Ⓔ medial tibial plateau, Ⓕ medial meniscus, Ⓖ medial collateral ligament, Ⓗ medial femoral condyle.

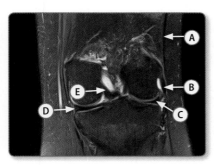

Figure 7.6 Coronal STIR magnetic resonance imaging of the left knee. Ⓐ Iliotibial band, Ⓑ lateral collateral ligament, Ⓒ lateral meniscus (posterior horn), Ⓓ medial meniscus (posterior horn), Ⓔ posterior cruciate ligament.

Imaging points

- No more than 5 mm of tibial condyle should be visible beyond a vertical line drawn at the most lateral margin of the femoral condyle (**Figure 7.6**). Suspect a tibial plateau fracture if > 5 mm of tibial condyle can be seen.
- The fabella is a sesamoid bone occasionally seen in the lateral head of gastrocnemius. Do not mistake the fabella for a fracture or loose body.

7.2 Knee and tibial injuries

Injuries of the knee are commonly complex, involving both osseous and soft tissue components of the joint.

Key facts

- A fender or **bumper fracture** is a proximal tibial fracture caused by a direct blow to the anterior knee. The name derives from the common method of injury: a moving vehicle striking a person at the level of the knees. The lateral tibial plateau is most commonly involved (**Figure 7.7**).
- A **lipohaemarthosis** may be the only radiographic sign of an intra-articular fracture of the knee (**Figure 7.8**).
- Shearing forces on the joint predispose the femoral condyles to **osteochondral fractures**. Osteochondral fractures involve both bone and overlying articular cartilage. They may also dislodge and form loose bodies in the joint.
- A **Segond fracture** is an avulsion injury of the lateral tibial condyle. It is associated with anterior cruciate and medial meniscal tears (**Figure 7.9**). A Segond fracture is a severe knee injury because of the associated marked damage to soft tissue.
- The patella usually dislocates laterally and self-reduces. Radiographs tend to be normal, so formal evaluation with

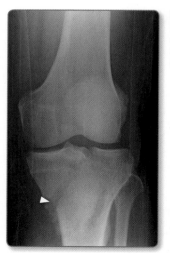

Figure 7.7 Anteroposterior radiograph of the left knee demonstrating an oblique proximal tibial fracture (arrowhead) with extension to the articular surface.

magnetic resonance imaging (MRI) is needed to confirm the extent of injury.

Radiological findings

Radiography Fractures of the knee are often difficult to identify because the fracture fragments are minimally displaced. Added

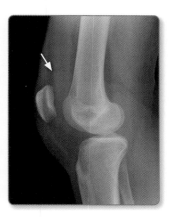

Figure 7.8 Lateral cross-table radiograph of the right knee (with horizontal X-ray beams parallel to the floor) demonstrating a horizontal fat-fluid level (due to a less dense upper layer of fat above the denser layer of blood).

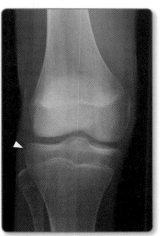

Figure 7.9 Anteroposterior radiograph of the right knee demonstrating a Segond fracture (arrowhead).

density across the bone suggests impaction and warrants further investigation.

Computerised tomography This imaging modality is used as an adjunct to assess the cortical integrity of the bones. Computerised tomography is also used for preoperative planning. It also provides a three-dimensional image of the fracture planes.

Magnetic resonance imaging This is the modality of choice for assessing ligamentous and meniscal injuries. MRI is also useful for assessing the sequelae of osteochondral injuries and patellar dislocations.

Key imaging findings

- To the inexperienced, a bipartite or multipartite patella may mimic a fracture. Remember that fractures have sharp margins (**Figure 7.10**).
- Non-uniform linear sclerosis in the tibial condyle is a subtle sign of an impacted fracture.
- Loss of the smooth cortical outline of the femoral condyles may be the only sign of an osteochondral fracture.

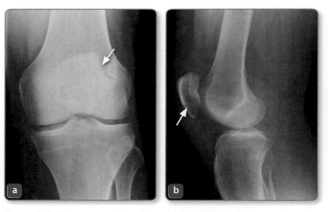

Figure 7.10 (a) Anteroposterior radiograph of the left knee demonstrating bipartite patella (arrow). (b) Lateral radiograph demonstrating fracture of the inferior pole of the patella (arrow).

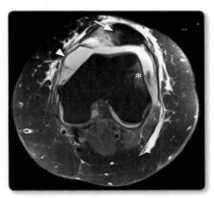

Figure 7.11 Axial MRI STIR of the left knee demonstrating 'kissing' contusions of the medial half of the patella (arrow) and lateral tibial plateau (*). There is a disrupted medial retinacular ligament injury (arrowhead) associated with joint effusion.

- Treat a thin sliver of bone adjacent to the lateral tibial condyle, no matter how small or subtle, as a Segond fracture until proven otherwise.
- Patellar dislocations show bone marrow oedema in the medial patellar facet and lateral femoral condyles on MRI (**Figure 7.11**). Bone marrow oedema occurs when the patella dislocates laterally and the medial patellar facet strikes the lateral femoral condyle, producing the characteristic appearance on MRI of 'kissing' contusions.

Treatment

Complex tibial plateau fractures usually need preoperative characterisation with computerised tomography and subsequent surgical management. Orthopaedic referral is crucial in complex knee injuries because of the associated soft tissue injuries. If untreated, long-term damage is possible.

7.3 Meniscal pathology

The medial and lateral menisci act as shock absorbers to help distribute force in the knee joint. Traumatic injury or degenerative wear can cause meniscal tears. Meniscal tears are classified as shown in **Table 7.1**.

Tear	Description
Vertical	A tear along the longitudinal axis of the meniscus (**Figure 7.12**)
Bucket handle	A complete longitudinal tear resulting in peripheral and inner fragments; the so-called bucket handle can lie beneath the posterior cruciate ligament, creating the double posterior cruciate ligament sign (**Figure 7.13**)
Radial	A tear in the circumferential fibres (**Figure 7.12b**)
Horizontal	A transverse tear along the horizontal axis of the meniscus (**Figure 7.12a**). A cleavage tear results from a complete transverse tear separating the superior and inferior fragments
Parrot's beak	A combined, incomplete radial and longitudinal tear

Table 7.1 Classification of meniscal tears

Key facts
- Meniscal tears can cause joint line pain, swelling, reduced range of motion and locking (if a displaced fragment is present).
- Tears may lead to degenerative arthropathic changes.

Radiological findings

Magnetic resonance imaging This is the modality of choice for identifying and classifying meniscal tears. To constitute a tear, the increased signal must extend to the surface of the meniscus. If the tear is in the anterior or posterior meniscal root, the meniscal body is usually subluxed.

Key imaging findings
- High signal extends to the joint surface.
- A ghostly meniscus is visible or the meniscus is displaced and therefore absent.
- The double posterior cruciate ligament sign is present (**Figure 7.13**).
- Parameniscal cysts are cystic structures arising from horizontal tears or degenerative meniscus. Cystic signal with associated communication is visible.

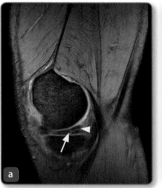
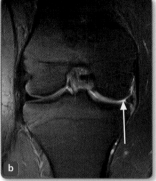

Figure 7.12 (a) Sagittal and (b) coronal T2-weighted magnetic resonance imaging of the right knee, showing horizontal (arrowhead), vertical (short arrow) and radial (long arrow) tears of the medial meniscus.

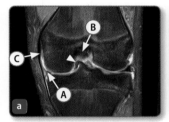
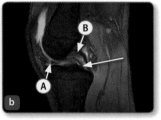

Figure 7.13 (a) Sagittal and (b) coronal T2-weighted magnetic resonance imaging of the right knee, showing a bucket handle tear (arrowhead) of the medial meniscus Ⓐ. The posterior cruciate ligament Ⓑ is seen on both views. The double posterior cruciate ligament PCL sign (long arrow) is visible on the sagittal view. Ⓒ Medial collateral ligament.

Treatment

Initial treatment with rest, ice, compression and elevation is useful. Large or symptomatic tears, or tears involving the meniscal roots, may need arthroscopic repair or excision.

7.4 Anterior cruciate ligament tears

The anterior cruciate ligament is injured when a traumatic force is applied to the knee in a twisting movement. Tears can be incomplete or complete.

Key facts

- Injuries of the anterior cruciate ligament are more common than injuries of the posterior cruciate ligament. Posterior cruciate ligament injuries usually happen only in road traffic accidents.
- Associated injuries of the posterolateral corner involve the lateral collateral ligament complex.

Radiological findings

Radiography Indirect evidence of an anterior cruciate ligament tear includes a Segond fracture (a fracture of the lateral tibial plateau) and a deep lateral notch. A deep lateral notch is produced by impaction of the lateral femoral condyle against the posterolateral tibial plateau.

Children may have an avulsion fracture of the tibial attachment.

Magnetic resonance imaging This is the modality of choice for anterior cruciate ligament tears. In acute injuries, ligamentous discontinuity and associated high signal on fluid-sensitive sequences are present (**Figure 7.14**). The ligament is more conspicuous after a few weeks, once the haemorrhage and oedema have subsided. Chronic tears can be difficult to interpret because scarring can make the torn ligament appear intact.

Tibial anterior translation of > 7 mm can make the posterior cruciate ligament appear to buckle and indicates an anterior cruciate ligament tear.

Key imaging findings

- A Segond fracture and deep lateral notch (or sulcus) sign may be visible (**Figure 7.15**).

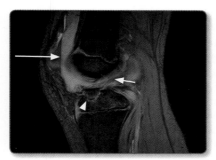

Figure 7.14 Sagittal T2-weighted magnetic resonance imaging of the right knee, showing anterior cruciate ligament disruption (short arrow) with avulsion of the tibial spine (arrowhead). The anterior cruciate ligament tear has caused lipohaemarthrosis with fat–blood interface present (long arrow).

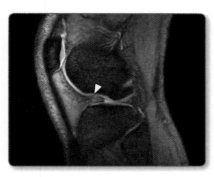

Figure 7.15 Sagittal T2-weighted magnetic resonance imaging of the right knee, showing a deep lateral notch (arrowhead) in the lateral femoral condyle. This results from tibial plateau impaction and is an indirect sign of an anterior cruciate ligament injury.

- Incomplete or complete ligamentous disruption is present.
- The degree of ligamentous oedema depends on the age of the injury.
- There is anterior tibial translation of > 7 mm.
- Bone bruising is visible on the lateral femoral condyle and the posterolateral tibial plateau.

Treatment

A conservative approach is appropriate for tears of the anterior cruciate ligament. Physiotherapy strengthens the quadriceps to stabilise the knee. Surgical repair involves anterior cruciate ligament reattachment for avulsion fractures or graft replacement for chronic tears.

7.5 Medial collateral ligament injuries

The medial collateral ligament has a superficial portion and a deep portion. The deep portion blends with the knee joint capsule, which is attached to the medial meniscus.

Isolated injuries typically occur with pure valgus stress without rotatory component, as in skiing injuries.

Tears of the medial collateral ligament are classified according to a universal grading system for ligamentous injuries (see p.28 and **Table 7.2**). **Figures 7.16–7.18** show different grades of tear.

Key facts

- The medial collateral ligament is extra-articular, so an accompanying knee effusion indicates associated internal derangement.
- Complete avulsions can occur in high-energy trauma.
- O'Donoghue's unhappy triad comprises an anterior cruciate ligament tear, a medial collateral ligament tear and a medial meniscal tear. The lateral compartmental is usually bruised as a result of valgus strain with rotation.

Radiological findings

Magnetic resonance imaging A bursa surrounded by fibrofatty tissue separates the superficial and deep portions. The superficial and deep portions are apparent as parallel dark bands.

Grade	Description and appearance on magnetic resonance imaging
1	Intact; low-signal band with perifascicular oedema
2	Partial tear with diffuse intrasubstance signal heterogeneity
3	Complete tear with loss of continuity

Table 7.2 Classification of tears of the medial collateral ligament

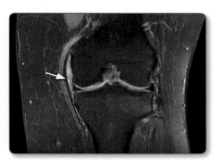

Figure 7.16 Coronal T2-weighted magnetic resonance imaging of the left knee, showing a grade 1 medial collateral ligament sprain (arrowhead). Perifascicular fluid is visible (arrow).

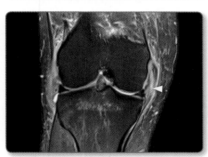

Figure 7.17 Coronal T2-weighted magnetic resonance imaging of the right knee, showing a grade 2 medial collateral ligament partial-thickness tear (arrowhead). There are diffuse intrasubstance signal changes.

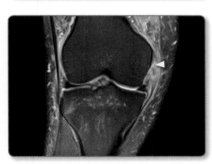

Figure 7.18 Coronal T2-weighted magnetic resonance imaging of the right knee, showing a grade 3 full-thickness tear (arrowhead) of the medial collateral ligament. Discontinuity of the ligament can be seen.

Key imaging findings

- Associated bony injuries include lateral contusions caused by valgus impaction, as well as medial avulsion injuries at femoral or tibial attachments.

- Meniscocapsular separation is visible when fluid is present between the medial meniscus and the capsule.

Treatment

Most injuries of the medial collateral ligament heal spontaneously. Therefore the aim of imaging is to identify other associated injuries. Grade 3 tears usually need immobilisation in a long-leg cast for ≥ 6 weeks.

7.6 Quadriceps tendon injuries

The extensor mechanism of the knee comprises the quadriceps muscle and tendon and the patella and patellar tendon. Quadriceps tendons are usually torn at musculotendinous junctions. Injuries can be acute or chronic, and tears can be partial or complete (see p.32).

Key facts

- Patients present with anterior knee pain and loss of active extension of the knee.
- Haematoma or haemarthrosis may mask clinical evidence of a tear.
- Quadriceps tendon tears are uncommon in the absence of pre-existing tendinopathy, which may be asymptomatic.
- Tears usually occur at musculotendinous junctions.
- If the patellar tendon appears corrugated on sagittal images, tensile strength is reduced. Therefore assess the patella and quadriceps with care to avoid converting a partial tear into a complete tear.

Radiological findings

Radiography The normal outline of the quadriceps is lost. The retracted tendon is visible as a mass of soft tissue. Calcification may be seen in chronic cases. Associated dense effusion may also be present.

Ultrasound This is the primary initial investigation in the acute setting for injuries to the quadriceps. Ultrasound is used to differentiate between partial and complete tears. Chronic tears may be difficult to distinguish in the presence of scar tissue.

Magnetic resonance imaging This is useful in chronic cases to distinguish scar tissue. MRI can be used to help identify associated features such as muscle belly atrophy and transient dislocation of the patella.

Key imaging findings
- Acute strain of the quadriceps tendon shows characteristic high-signal fluid intensity.
- In a partial tear, there is a focal defect of the tendon, hypoechoicity on ultrasound and increased internal signal on MRI.
- In a complete tear, there is focal discontinuity of the tendon, with the gap filled with haemorrhagic fluid.
- A diagnosis of haematoma is based on typical characteristics according to age (see p.34).

Treatment
Complete tears need reapposition of the discountinuous margins. This can be done either conservatively or surgically. With the conservative approach, ultrasound can help determine any potential gap.

7.7 Osgood–Schlatter disease

Osgood–Schlatter disease can present in various ways but the common feature is patellar tendon abnormality. The abnormality usually, but not always, includes an osseous component. Persistent ossific fragments are often found in a thickened patellar tendon in the later stages of the disease.

Key facts
- Osgood–Schlatter disease is five times more likely to affect males, usually boys aged 10–15 years. The disease is bilateral in 25% of cases.
- The cause is unknown, but trauma (acute or chronic) may play a role. There is usually a history of recent athletic activity.

- The disease has five stages based on its appearance on MRI: normal, early, progressive, terminal and healing.

> ## Clinical insight
>
> Osgood–Schlatter disease is part of a family of osteochondrosis diseases. The family includes **Sinding-Larsen–Johansson syndrome** (affecting the proximal patellar tendon and the inferior margin of the patella), **Sever's disease** (calcaneal apophysis), **Köhler's disease** (affecting the navicular bone), **Freiberg's disease** (affecting the foot metatarsal), **Panner's disease** (affecting the capitellum), **Kienböck's disease** (affecting the lunate) and **Scheuermann's disease** (affecting the thoracic spine).

Radiological findings

Radiography Ossific fragments of the tibial tuberosity ossification centre are visible. Pretibial soft tissue swelling may be present.

Ultrasound Look for patellar tendinopathy with fragmentation of the ossification centre. Associated infrapatellar bursitis may be present.

Magnetic resonance imaging There is increased T1 and T2 signal at the tibial insertion site. This finding reflects the presence of blood products (on T1-weighted MRI) and oedema (on T2-weighted MRI) in the acute stages.

Associated pretibial high signal and deep infrapatellar bursitis may be present. Fragmentation and separation of ossification centres may lead to partial avulsion and proximal retraction on follow-up scans.

Key imaging findings

- Features of tendinopathy (see p.32) are visible at the distal attachment of the patellar tendon.
- An opened shell shape is seen if there is a tear and widening in the ossification centre.
- A high signal on short T1 inversion recovery MRI differentiates an avulsed, fractured fragment from a physiologically ununited secondary ossification centre.

Treatment

Conservative management with immobilisation and rest leads to recovery in most cases.

7.8 Baker's cyst

A Baker's cyst, also known as a popliteal cyst, is caused by over-accumulation of synovial fluid in a bursa on the posterior aspect of the knee. The term cyst is a misnomer because this synovial-lined cavity communicates with the knee joint.

Key facts
- A Baker's cyst is usually asymptomatic. It presents as an asymmetric cosmetic deformity on the back of the knee.
- It may arise secondary to regional inflammation or an intra-articular cartilaginous tear.
- Patients may remember feeling a pop in the back of the knee, followed by calf pain. This history indicates a rupture. A ruptured Baker's cyst causes a painful, swollen calf, often mimicking deep venous thrombosis.

Radiological findings

Ultrasound A Baker's cyst appears as a well-defined anechoic mass with posterior acoustic enhancement. Baker's cysts occasionally have complex imaging features, such as thin internal septations and small mobile echogenic debris. No internal vascularity is present on Doppler studies, which are a useful adjunct to exclude a popliteal artery aneurysm.

Magnetic resonance imaging Baker's cysts are a common incidental finding on MRI of the knee done for other clinical indications. They manifest as well-demarcated cystic masses of homogeneous fluid intensity (high T2 signal, low T1 signal).

An interdigitated neck-like structure is commonly visualised between the medial head of the gastrocnemius and the semimembranosus muscle tendons. This structure represents communication of the bursa with the joint (**Figure 7.19**).

Key imaging findings
- Baker's cysts are anechoic on ultrasound.
- They are avascular.
- A fluid signal is found on MRI (high T2 signal, low T1 signal; **Figure 7.20**)

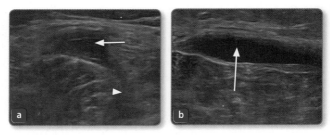

Figure 7.19 Ultrasound of the knee. (a) Transverse view demonstrating a Baker's cyst (arrow) communicating with the knee joint (arrowhead). (b) Longitudinal view demonstrating fluid collection (arrow) superficial to the gastrocnemius, consistent with rupture of a Baker's cyst.

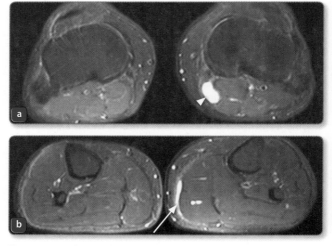

Figure 7.20 Axial T2-weighted magnetic resonance imaging of the knees. (a) A Baker's cyst (arrowhead) is visible in the left knee. (b) A more distal section shows ruptured fluid collection (arrow) superficial to the medial gastrocnemius.

Treatment

Most Baker's cysts need no treatment, but symptomatic cysts may be aspirated. Surgical resection is reserved for debilitating lesions that do not respond to corticosteroid injection.

Foot and ankle

8.1 Key anatomy

The ankle comprises the tibiotalar joint, the subtalar joint and the inferior tibiofibular joint (**Figures 8.1** and **8.2**). Three groups of tendons pass the ankle joint: one anteriorly, one posteriorly and one laterally. In the anterior group are the tendons of the extensor digitorum longus, extensor hallucis longus and tibialis anterior, which pass under the flexor retinaculum. In the posterior group are the tendons of tibialis posterior, flexor digitorum longus and flexor hallucis longus, which pass under the flexor retinaculum. In the lateral group are the tendons of the peroneus brevis (anterior) and peroneus longus.

The ankle is supported medially by the deltoid ligament and laterally by the lateral ligament complex. The lateral ligament

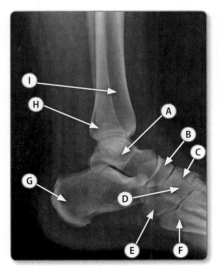

Figure 8.1 Lateral radiograph of the left ankle. (A) Talus, (B) navicular, (C) intermediate cuneiform, (D) lateral cuneiform, (E) cuboid, (F) 5th metatarsal, (G) calcaneus, (H) fibula, (I) tibia.

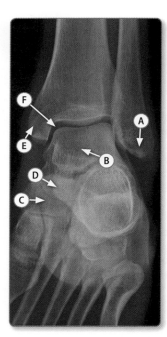

Figure 8.2 Anteroposterior radiograph of the left ankle. (A) Lateral malleolus, (B) talus, (C) navicular, (D) sustentaculum tali of calcaneus, (E) medial malleolus, (F) ankle joint.

complex consists of three ligaments: the anterior and posterior talofibular ligaments and the calcaneofibular ligament (**Figure 8.3** and **8.4**).

In the foot, the Lisfranc ligament attaches the medial cuneiform to the 2nd metatarsal. In a normal anteroposterior radiograph of the foot, the 2nd metatarsal aligns with the intermediate cuneiform (**Figure 8.5**). In an oblique radiograph, the 3rd metatarsal aligns with the lateral cuneiform (**Figure 8.6**).

Key facts

- On the anteroposterior mortise view of the ankle, the joint space should be equal all the way round.
- The distance between the distal tibia and fibula should be ≤ 6 mm at the point 1 cm above the tibiotalar joint. Widening suggests syndesmotic injury.

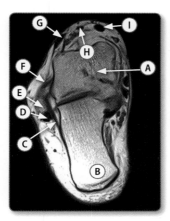

Figure 8.3 Axial T1-weighted magnetic resonance imaging of the right ankle below the tibiotalar joint. (A) Talus, (B) calcaneus, (C) calcaneofibular ligament, (D) peroneus longus and peroneus brevis tendons, (E) distal fibula, (F) anterior talofibular ligament, (G) extensor digitorum longus tendon, (H) extensor hallucis longus tendon, (I) tibialis anterior tendon.

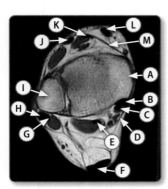

Figure 8.4 Axial T1-weighted magnetic resonance imaging of the right ankle above the tibiotalar joint. (A) Medial malleolus, (B) tibialis posterior tendon, (C) flexor digitorum longus tendon, (D) flexor retinaculum, (E) flexor hallucis longus tendon, (F) Achilles tendon, (G) peroneus brevis tendon, (H) peroneus longus tendon, (I) lateral malleolus, (J) extensor digitorum longus tendon, (K) extensor hallucis longus tendon, (L) tibialis anterior tendon, (M) extensor retinaculum.

- Bohler's angle is the angle between a line drawn from the upper edge of the calcaneal body to the articular facet at the subtalar joint and a line drawn from this facet to the upper edge of the anterior process of the calcaneus. Bohler's angle is normally 20–40°. A decreased Bohler's angle suggests fracture of the calcaneus.
- Do not mistake non-fused ossification centres for fractures. Typical locations for non-fused ossification centres include the distal end of the fibula (os fibularis), the margin of the

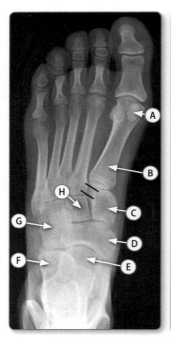

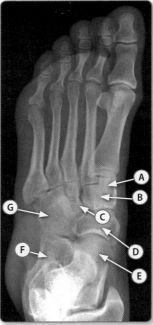

Figure 8.5 Anteroposterior radiograph of the left foot, showing the location of the Lisfranc ligament (hyphenated lines). (A) Sesamoid bone in the tendon of flexor hallucis longus, (B) 1st metatarsal, (C) medial cuneiform, (D) navicular, (E) talus, (F) calcaneus, (G) cuboid, (H) intermediate cuneiform.

Figure 8.6 Oblique radiograph of the left foot. (A) Medial cuneiform, (B) intermediate cuneiform, (C) lateral cuneiform, (D) navicular, (E) talus, (F) calcaneus, (G) cuboid.

navicular (os navicularis) and posterior to the body of the talus (os trigonum).

8.2 Ankle injuries

Ankle injuries are common. They are frequently investigated in the accident and emergency department.

Key facts
- The Weber classification is used to define and assess the severity of ankle fractures (**Table 8.1**). Fractures are classified according to the level of distal fibula fracture in relation to the ankle mortise.
- A bimalleolar fracture is a fracture of both the medial and lateral malleolus. A trimalleolar fracture further involves the posterior surface of the distal tibia.

Radiological findings

Radiography Linear lucencies, cortical breech and displaced fracture fragments are the predominant radiographic findings in ankle fractures.

Computerised tomography This is used as an adjunct for presurgical management of complex fractures. Computerised tomography provides the most detail for osseous fracture planes and cortical involvement.

Key imaging findings
- Non-uniformity of the joint space of the ankle mortise on an anteroposterior radiograph indicates talar shift and instability of the ankle. Surgery is needed to avoid premature degeneration of the ankle joint.
- A **Maisonneuve fracture** is a spiral fracture of the proximal fibula (**Figure 8.10**). This type of fracture is usually associated

Grade	Description
A	Fracture of the tip of the lateral malleolus below the level of the ankle mortise: stable (**Figure 8.7**)
B	Spiral or oblique fracture at the level of the ankle mortise and distal tibiofibular syndesmosis: stable or unstable (**Figure 8.8**)
C	Fracture proximal to the distal tibiofibular syndesmosis: unstable (**Figure 8.9**)

Table 8.1 Weber classification of ankle fractures

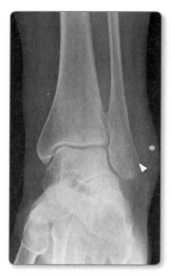

Figure 8.7 Anteroposterior radiograph of the left ankle, showing an undisplaced lateral malleolar fracture (arrowhead) with associated swelling of the lateral soft tissue (*).

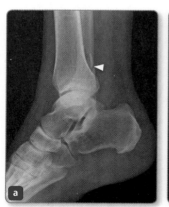

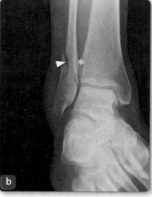

Figure 8.8 (a) Lateral and (b) anteroposterior radiographs of the right ankle, showing an oblique lateral malleolar fracture (arrowhead) at the level of the syndesmosis (*).

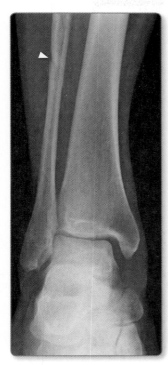

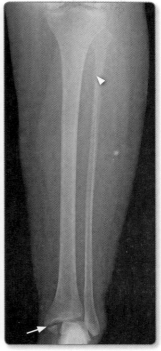

Figure 8.9 Anteroposterior radiograph of the right ankle, showing a spiral fracture of the fibular shaft (arrowhead) proximal to the syndesmosis.

Figure 8.10 Anteroposterior radiograph of the left tibia, showing a Maisonneuve fracture (i.e. a spiral fracture of the proximal fibular shaft; arrowhead). There is an associated fracture of the transverse medial malleolus (arrow).

with instability of the ankle mortise. The fibular fracture is easily missed or overlooked because of its proximity to the knee.

- A **Tillaux fracture** is a type 3 Salter–Harris injury of the lateral aspect of the distal tibial epiphysis with varying degrees of displacement (**Figure 8.11**).

- A **pilon fracture** involves the supramalleolar aspect of the distal tibia. This type of fracture extends into the ankle mortise (**Figure 8.12**).
- A **triplane fracture** is a paediatric injury with three individual fracture planes (**Figure 8.13**):
  - vertical fracture of the epiphysis
  - horizontal fracture across the physis
  - oblique fracture of the metaphysis

Treatment

Talar shift indicates ankle instability, which needs open reduction and internal fixation. All type C Weber injuries are treated surgically. For type B Weber injuries, use discretion to decide

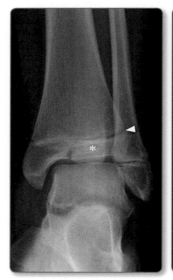
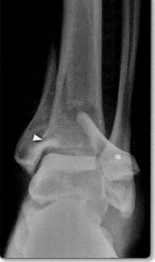

Figure 8.11 Anteroposterior radiograph of the left ankle, showing a Tillaux fracture involving the lateral portion (*), which shows slight displacement with separation of the epiphysis laterally (arrowhead).

Figure 8.12 Anteroposterior radiograph of the left ankle, showing a pilon fracture: split distal fragments (*) and shortening and impaction (arrowhead) caused by a distal tibial fracture with intra-articular extension.

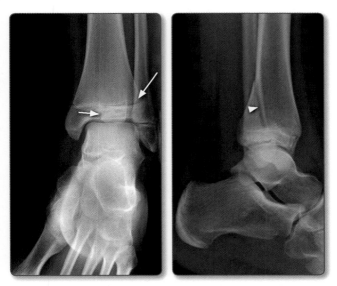

Figure 8.13 Anteroposterior and lateral radiographs of the left ankle, showing a triplane fracture. The triplane fracture comprises a vertical fracture of the epiphysis (short arrow), a horizontal fracture across the physis (long arrow) and an oblique fracture of the metaphysis (arrowhead).

whether surgery is needed. Type A Weber fractures are treated conservatively.

For Tillaux, pilon and triplane fractures, preoperative computerised tomography is helpful.

8.3 Foot injuries

The foot is commonly injured in athletes and in cases involving a high axial loading force, such as landing on the feet after jumping from a great height.

Key facts

- When jumpers land on their feet, the calcaneus is the first bone to sustain the loading force. A fracture, commonly comminuted, may result (**Figure 8.14**).

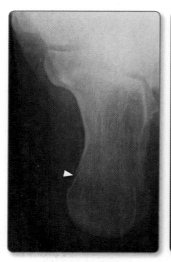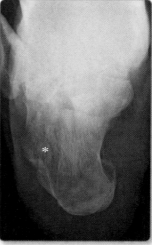

Figure 8.14 Anteroposterior radiographs of the foot, showing (a) left undisplaced fracture (arrowhead) and (b) right comminuted displaced fracture (*) of the calcaneus in different patients.

- A fracture of the base of the 5th metatarsal is an inversion injury that can mimic an ankle fracture (**Figure 8.15**).
- A dancer's or **Jones fracture** is a fracture of the proximal diaphysis of the 5th metatarsal. This type of fracture is predisposed to non-union (**Figure 8.16**).
- The **Lisfranc injury** is the most common dislocation of the foot. This injury is the dorsal dislocation of the tarsometatarsal joints secondary to disruption of the Lisfranc ligament (**Figure 8.17**).
- Stress fractures of the foot, also known as **march fractures**, occur in marathon runners and military personnel. These fractures commonly involve the calcaneus or the metatarsals (**Figure 8.18**).

Radiological findings

Radiography Misalignment of the 2nd metatarsal and the intermediate cuneiform, and of the 3rd metatarsal and the lateral

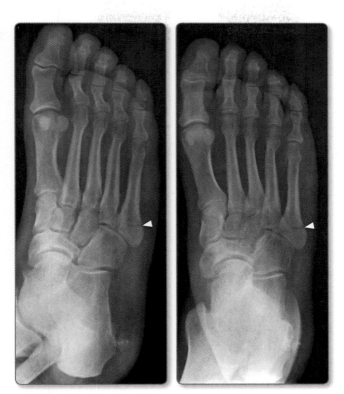

Figure 8.15 Oblique and anteroposterior radiographs of the left foot, showing an avulsion fracture of the base of the 5th metatarsal (arrowheads).

cuneiform, is the hallmark of a Lisfranc injury. Stress fractures occur over time and present radiographically as ill-defined added density of the affected bone, with possible overlying periosteal reaction.

Computerised tomography Cross-sectional imaging helps visualise small associated fracture fragments in Lisfranc injuries.

Magnetic resonance imaging Although not used in the acute trauma setting, magnetic resonance imaging (MRI) is helpful

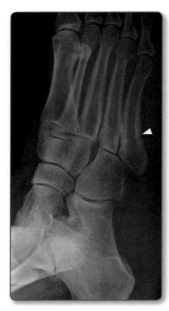
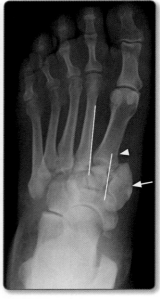

Figure 8.16 Oblique radiograph of the left foot, showing a dancer's or Jones fracture of the proximal diaphysis of the 5th metatarsal (arrowhead). The fracture is extra-articular.

Figure 8.17 Anteroposterior radiograph of the right foot, showing a Lisfranc injury. The injury involves loss of alignment between the 2nd metatarsal and the intermediate cuneiform (solid lines). There is also homolateral displacement (arrowhead) of the 1st to 5th metatarsals. Associated fractures of the medial (arrow) and intermediate cuneiform are present.

when diagnosing stress fractures that are indeterminate on radiograph. Stress fractures show bone marrow oedema and localised periostitis. Lisfranc ligament and soft tissue injuries are also better seen on MRI.

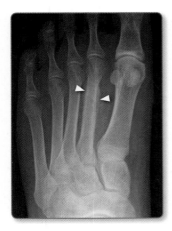

Figure 8.18 Anteroposterior radiograph of the right foot, showing the fluffy appearance of the periosteum (arrowheads) at the site of a stress fracture of the 2nd metatarsal shaft.

Key imaging findings

- The metatarsals are displaced laterally in Lisfranc injuries.
  - In a divergent Lisfranc injury, the 2nd to 5th metatarsals are displaced; the 1st metatarsal remains neutral or displaces medially.
  - In a homolateral Lisfranc injury, the 1st to 5th metatarsals are displaced.
- Midfoot fractures are commonly associated with Lisfranc injuries.
- The fluffy appearance of the affected bone, caused by its increased density, is key to identifying stress fractures.

Treatment

Lisfranc injuries must be treated surgically. Without timely management, the midfoot could collapse entirely.

8.4 Achilles tendon pathology

The Achilles tendon is the thickest and strongest tendon. However, it is the tendon most frequently injured. It is enclosed in a paratenon, a thin film of connective tissue, rather than a synovial sheath. Pathologies of the Achilles tendon can be acute or chronic.

Key facts

- Achilles tendinopathy presents with pain, usually during exercise. However, the pain can be persistent and occur even without exercise in chronic cases.
- Tears of the Achilles tendon may be spontaneous or secondary to trauma. Patients often describe feeling and hearing the tendon suddenly snap.
- Anatomical variants are:
  - the plantaris tendon coursing medial to the Achilles tendon
  - the accessory soleus muscle lying between the Achilles tendon posteriorly and the flexor hallucis longus anteriorly (and often mistaken for a space-occupying lesion)
  - Haglund's syndrome, caused by thickening of the distal tendon resulting from chronic irritation from the heel cup of a shoe.

Radiological findings

Ultrasound   Patients are scanned prone, with their feet hanging off the edge of the table. This position allows dynamic movement. Hypoechoic regions indicate tendinopathy (see p.28). Neovascularisation may be present (**Figure 8.19**). Tears appear as partial or complete discontinuity of the echogenic fibres (**Figure 8.20**).

Magnetic resonance imaging   Hypertrophy and loss of anterior concavity indicate tendinopathy. Tears show fibre discontinuity, appearing as intervening high-signal areas on T2-weighted images (**Figure 8.21**).

Key imaging findings

- The tendon is thickened (anteroposterior diameter, > 6 mm) in tendinopathy.

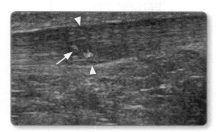

Figure 8.19 Longitudinal ultrasound of the Achilles tendon, showing fusiform hypertrophy of the mid portion of the tendon (between the arrowheads). The areas of hypoechoicity are tendinopathy (arrow), with Doppler flow indicating neovascularisation. These findings are consistent with tendinitis.

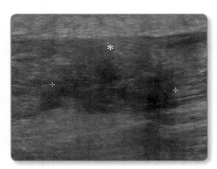

Figure 8.20 Longitudinal ultrasound of the Achilles tendon, showing discontinuous tendon fibres (between the + signs) in the deeper portion; the superficial fibres (*) are intact.

- Anterior concavity is lost, so the tendon becomes flat or convex.
- There may be associated retrocalcaneal bursitis.
- Tears usually occur 2–6 cm proximal to the insertion, in the so-called zone of vulnerability.

Treatment
Persistent tendinopathy can improve with eccentric physiotherapy exercises. A plaster cast in the equinus position or surgical repair may be

Clinical insight

The maximum tendon gap with the ankle in full plantar flexion on ultrasound is an important measurement when deciding how to manage the pathology.

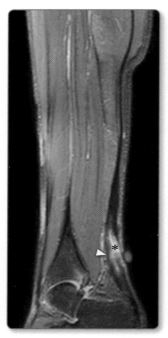

Figure 8.21 Sagittal short T1 inversion recovery magnetic resonance imaging of the right calf, showing focal haematoma (*) in a partial tear of the Achilles tendon, with discontinuity of superficial layers but intact deeper fibres (arrowhead).

indicated, depending on the degree of tear and the length of the gap with the ankle in plantar flexion.

8.5 Tibialis posterior dysfunction

Tibialis posterior dysfunction is a complex progressive condition. It presents in various ways, from tendinopathy to tendinitis to tears. A common presentation is pain and swelling in the medial hindfoot. Function is progressively lost because of acquired pes planus.

Key fact

- Tibialis posterior dysfunction occurs in women aged 40–60 years. Risk factors include diabetes, rheumatoid arthritis and obesity.

Radiological findings

Radiography Abnormal features of progressive pes planus, heel valgus and degenerative arthropathy may be present.

Ultrasound Tendon thickening and inhomogeneity with hypoechoic areas are present on ultrasound (**Figure 8.22**). The discontinuity in tendon tears is most apparent on longitudinal views (**Figure 8.23**).

> ### Clinical insight
>
> The so-called too-many-toes sign indicates tibialis posterior dysfunction. More toes than usual are visible when the foot is viewed from behind the patient. The sign is caused by the foot pointing out more laterally.

Magnetic resonance imaging Partial tears can split longitudinally along the tendon, resulting in thickening and heterogeneous signal intensity (**Figure 8.24**).

Key imaging findings
- The tendon sheath may remain intact even with a full-thickness tear of the tendon. The sheath collapses when

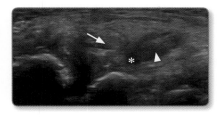

Figure 8.22 Transverse ultrasound of the medial ankle, showing the tibialis posterior tendon. The tendon contains areas of hypoechoicity (arrowhead), and there is increased fluid in the tendon sheath (*). These findings are consistent with tenosynovitis. The adjacent flexor digitorum longus (arrow) is normal by comparison.

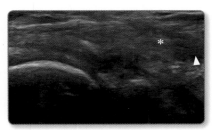

Figure 8.23 Longitudinal ultrasound of the medial ankle, showing a thickened hypoechoic tibialis posterior tendon end (*) with a tendon gap (arrowhead). These findings are consistent with a degenerative tear.

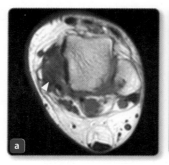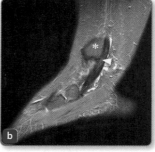

Figure 8.24 (a) Axial T1-weighted and (b) sagittal short T1 inversion recovery magnetic resonance imaging of the left ankle, showing a longitudinal split (arrowheads) in a hypertrophied tibialis posterior tendon posterior to the medial malleolus (*). There is increased fluid in the tendon sheath.

the tendon retracts on dynamic plantar flexion of the foot.
- Associated sinus tarsi collapse or anterior talofibular ligament tears can be present on MRI.

Treatment
Tendinopathies are treated conservatively. However, tears may need to be repaired surgically to prevent long-term flatfoot deformity.

8.6 Morton's neuroma

A non-neoplastic fusiform swelling of the digital nerve is called a Morton's neuroma, although it is not a neuroma but a perineural fibrosis. Morton's neuroma occurs in the intermetatarsal (web) space. Patients present with pain, numbness or both, in the contiguous halves of two toes.

Key facts
- The intermetatarsal spaces most commonly involved are the 2nd and 3rd (**Figure 8.25**).

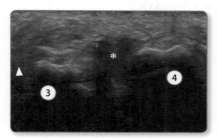

Figure 8.25 Axial ultrasound of the web space between the 3rd ③ and 4th ④ metatarsal heads. The well-defined hypoechoic lesion (*) is consistent with a Morton's neuroma. Its hypoechoicity contrasts with the echoic fat in the adjacent web space (arrowhead).

- Differential diagnosis includes capsulitis or bursitis of the metatarsophalangeal joints, ganglions and nerve sheath tumours, as well as other causes of metatarsalgia.
- Morton's neuroma is commoner in women aged 30–50 years.

Radiological findings

Radiography This is not useful, except to exclude other causes of metatarsalgia, such as metatarsophalangeal arthropathy or stress fractures.

Ultrasound This is the investigation of choice. However, like many procedures, its usefulness is operator-dependent.

Magnetic resonance imaging Morton's neuroma appears on MRI as a bulbous mass arising between the metatarsal heads. The lesions typically have low-signal intensity on T1- and T2-weighted images.

Key imaging findings

- Ultrasound shows a hypoechoic lesion between the distal intermetatarsal spaces (**Figure 8.26**). Dynamic side-to-side squeezing of the metatarsal heads can produce a visible so-called Mulder's click.
- Morton's neuromas are highly vascular, so the lesions are typically uniformly enhanced on MRI.

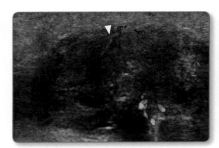

Figure 8.26 Longitudinal ultrasound showing the heterogeneous, mostly hypoechoic features of Morton's neuroma, with peripheral vascularisation (arrowhead) on Doppler flow.

Treatment

Patients sometimes obtain relief from the pain or numbness by simply changing footwear. Relief can be provided in most patients with local steroid injection, which may be done under ultrasound guidance. Persistent Morton's neuromas may need surgical excision.

8.7 Tarsal coalition

Tarsal coalition is the abnormal fibrous, cartilaginous or osseous union or two or more tarsal bones. If the coalition is osseous, the bony bar usually produces complete fusion by the age of 12 years.

Different types of tarsal coalition exist. The calcaneonavicular, talocalcaneal and talonavicular types are common. The calcaneocuboidal, cuboidalnavicular and navicular–cuneiform types are uncommon.

Key facts

- Tarsal coalition may be asymptomatic and an incidental finding.
- In children, the condition can present as a rigid flatfoot. The plantar arch forms at the age of 3–5 years.
- The associated features of peroneal tendinopathy or sinus tarsi syndrome may be the presenting complaint in undiagnosed coalitions.

Radiological findings

Radiography Weight-bearing anteroposterior and lateral radiographs can show key findings such as the C sign (**Figure 8.27**) and the anteater sign (**Figure 8.28**).

Computerised tomography Coronal reformats show the coalition well. Narrowing of the middle facet with sclerotic and cystic margins may be present in fibrous coalitions (**Figure 8.29a**). There may be abnormal downward sloping of the sustentaculum tali or a horizontally oriented middle facet articular surface. The extent of joint involvement and secondary bony changes in fibrous coalition are also seen on computerised tomography. Three-dimensional reconstruction can help surgical visualisation (**Figure 8.29b**).

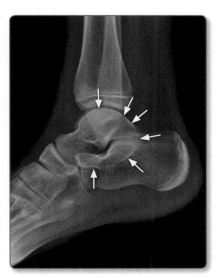

Figure 8.27 Weight-bearing lateral radiograph of the right ankle, showing the C sign (arrows) indicating talocalcaneal coalition.

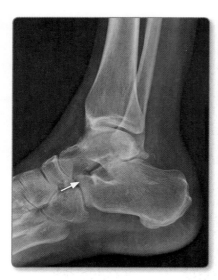

Figure 8.28 Weight-bearing lateral radiograph of the right ankle, showing the anteater sign. The prominent and broad tip of the anterior process (arrow) of the calcaneum resembles an anteater's nose. Calcaneonavicular coalition was confirmed on magnetic resonance imaging.

Bone scan In the region of the coalition, there is increased uptake that lacks specificity.

Magnetic resonance imaging This is used to differentiate osseous coalitions from non-osseous coalitions. The extent of joint involvement and secondary bony changes can also be seen on MRI. Coalitions may be an incidental finding during the investigation of ankle pain.

Key imaging findings
- Talar beaking, which arises from the dorsum of the head of the talus, is present in two-thirds of cases.
- The C sign indicates talocalcaneal coalition. A characteristic C-shaped line is created by the outline of the talar dome and the inferior margin of the sustentaculum tali on lateral radiographs.
- The anteater sign indicates calcaneonavicular coalition. The anterior process of the calcaneum is prominent and has a broad tip.

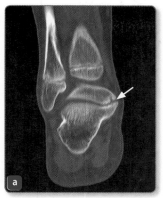

Figure 8.29 (a) Coronal computerised tomography of the left ankle, showing fibrous talocalcaneal coalition (arrow) with sclerotic and cystic margins at the narrowed middle facet articulation. (b) Three-dimensional computerised tomography used to help in surgical planning.

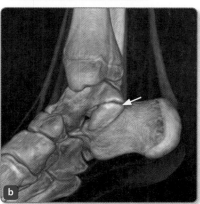

• The middle facet is not visible on a weight-bearing lateral radiograph of the ankle.

Treatment

Surgery is indicated if the condition is painful and the patient has limited function.

9.1 Key anatomy

The cervical spine is usually assessed by three projections: an anteroposterior, a lateral and an open-mouth odontoid peg view. The lateral projection should include the C7–T1 junction. Trace four lines when assessing the lateral projection (**Figure 9.1**); the lines should be smooth and without steps.

- Line A: anterior vertebral soft tissues. Anterior to C3 and above should be < 3 mm. Below C4, the soft tissue width can be ≤ 10 mm.
- Line B: anterior margins of the vertebral bodies.

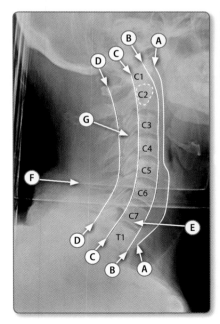

Figure 9.1 Lateral radiograph of the cervical spine. Ⓐ Anterior vertebral soft tissue line, Ⓑ anterior vertebral line, Ⓒ posterior vertebral line, Ⓓ spinolaminar line, Ⓔ vertebral body, Ⓕ spinous process, Ⓖ facet joint. Dashed line, Axis (or Harris) ring.

Radiological findings

- Axis (Harris) ring is at the base of C2 (**Figure 9.1**). It is a normal finding caused by a combination of overlapping bony structures. The ring is usually incomplete inferiorly. However, if it is disrupted elsewhere a fracture of the peg should be suspected.
- A thin black line may appear to run through the peg on the peg view. This is the Mach effect and results from overlapping shadows. Do not confuse this artefact for a fracture.
- Assess the paraspinal lines on the anteroposterior radiographs of the spine (**Figure 9.5**). Abnormal widening may indicate haematoma or collection.

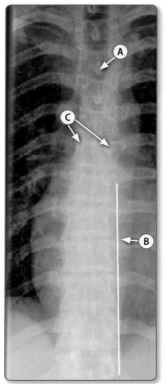

Figure 9.5 Anteroposterior radiograph of the thoracic spine. (A) Spinous process, (B) left paraspinal line, (C) pedicles.

- The pedicles should align with those above and below. The anteroposterior view of the vertebral body resembles an owl, with pedicles as the eyes and the spinous process as the beak. A winking owl with an absent pedicle can be a sign of bony destruction (see section 10.1, *Bone tumours*).

9.2 Atlantoaxial fractures

Clinical features of cervical spine trauma include neck pain or tenderness, focal neurological deficit and paraesthesia in the extremities. Various mechanisms of injury can result in various types of spinal fractures (**Table 9.1**).

Imaging helps when deciding if a fracture is stable or unstable. Simple wedge fractures and spinous process fractures are stable. Teardrop fractures, bilateral locked facets (section 9.4, *Facet injuries*), hangman's fractures and Jefferson fractures are unstable.

Key facts

- Cervical spine radiographs after trauma are unnecessary if the patient is fully conscious, is not intoxicated, has normal neurological status and has no neck pain or tenderness.
- Most serious cervical spine injuries are caused by road traffic collisions. A fall from a height of > 1 m can also cause serious injury.
- The C1–C2 and C5–C7 areas are most susceptible to trauma.

Mechanism of injury	Outcomes
Flexion	• Crush fracture • Fracture dislocations and ligament rupture • Teardrop fractures
Extension	• Odontoid peg fracture • Hangman's fracture • Anterior spinal artery occlusion
Vertical compression	• Atlas fracture • Burst fractures
Rotation	• Facet joint dislocations • Posterior column injury

Table 9.1 Mechanisms of injury and types of resulting spinal vertebral injury

Radiological findings

Radiography Carefully check the alignment of the cervical spine, including the odontoid peg (see section 9.1, *Key anatomy*, **Figures 9.1–9.3**). Open-mouth views are needed to identify odontoid peg fractures (**Figure 9.6a,b**).

Computerised tomography This is often done when the lateral cervical radiograph fails to visualise the C7–T1 level. Sagittal reconstruction allows accurate assessment of fractures for surgical planning (**Figure 9.6c,d**).

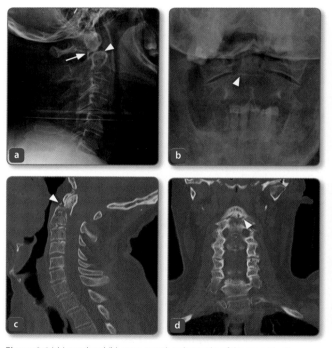

Figure 9.6 (a) Lateral and (b) open-mouth radiographs of the cervical spine. (c) Sagittal and (d) coronal computerised tomography is used to help surgical planning. An odontoid peg base fracture is present (arrowheads), with posterior displacement (arrow).

Magnetic resonance imaging For soft tissue injuries such as acute disc herniation, epidural haematoma and cord contusion, magnetic resonance imaging (MRI) is useful.

Key imaging findings

- A **Jefferson fracture** involves displacement of the lateral masses beyond the margins of C2 on the peg view (**Figure 9.7**). C1, being a ring, breaks in two or more places.
- In a **hangman's fracture**, the C2 posterior elements are fractured and C2 is displaced anterior to C3 (**Figure 9.8**). This fracture is caused by hyperextension and distraction, as in an injury involving a car dashboard.
- A **clay shoveller's fracture** is a spinous process fracture of C6 or C7 (**Figure 9.9**).
- A **teardrop fracture** is an anteroinferior cervical vertebral fracture caused by a spine flexion injury from vertical axial

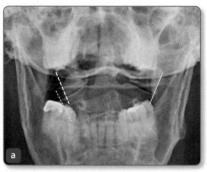

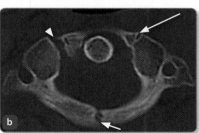

Figure 9.7 (a) Open-mouth radiograph of the cervical spine, showing malalignment between a C2 lateral mass on the right (thin dashed line) to the C1 lateral border (thick dashed line), consistent with a Jefferson fracture. Normal C1–C2 alignment is shown on the left (solid line). (b) Axial computerised tomography of C1, showing the displaced fracture on the right anteriorly (arrowhead), incomplete fracture on the left (long arrow), and midline fracture posteriorly (short arrow).

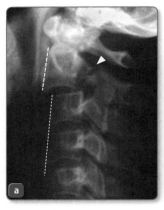
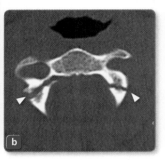

Figure 9.8 (a) Lateral radiograph of the cervical spine, showing a C1 posterior element fracture (arrowhead) with anterior displacement of C2 (thick dashed line) to C3 (thin dashed line). (b) Axial computerised tomography of C1, showing bilateral posterior process fractures (arrowheads).

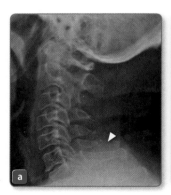
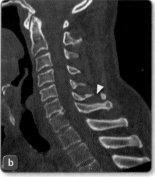

Figure 9.9 (a) Lateral radiograph of the cervical spine, showing a displaced spinous process fracture of C6 (arrowhead). (b) The fracture (arrowhead) is also visible on sagittal computerised tomography, which excluded other bony injuries.

compression (**Figure 9.10**). This type of fracture is typically associated with spinal cord injury caused by posterior vertebral retropulsion.

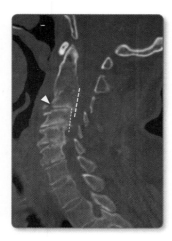

Figure 9.10 Sagittal computerised tomography showing a flexion teardrop fracture of a C3 vertebral body anteroinferiorly (arrowhead). Posterior C3 retropulsion (thick dashed line) in relation to the C4 vertebra below (thin dashed line) often results in underlying neurological injury.

Treatment

Stable fractures can be treated with a brace. Unstable injuries need surgical fixation or fusion.

9.3 Vertebral fractures

Thoracic and lumbar vertebral fractures are less common than cervical spine injuries. The thoracic spine has limited mobility and its fractures are generally stable. The lumbar spine has more mobility and is more prone to fracture.

Key facts

- Common causes of spinal fractures are osteoporosis, trauma and metastatic disease.
- The three basic fracture patterns are:
  - wedge (anterior height reduced)
  - biconcave (middle height reduced)
  - crush (posterior height reduced)
- Fractures can be graded in severity based on the degree of vertebral body height loss (**Figures 9.11** and **9.12**).
- Burst fractures caused by axial compression have retro-pulsed fragments that may cause neurological compromise.

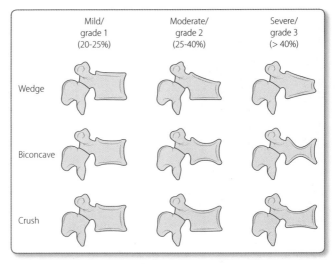

Figure 9.11 Grading of vertebral fractures

Clinical insight

A **Chance fracture** is a horizontal fracture of the vertebral body and posterior elements at T10–L2 (**Figure 9.13**). This is an unstable fracture with potential neurological injury. Chance fractures are usually caused by a seatbelt-related hyperflexion injury and are often associated with serious retroperitoneal injuries.

Radiological findings

Radiography The standard views are the anteroposterior and lateral radiographs (**Figure 9.14**). Burst fractures may show interpedicular widening on the anteroposterior view (**Figure 9.14a**).

Computerised tomography This is used to assess major trauma and unstable injuries. Computerised tomography (CT) can also be used to assess the degree of retropulsion in burst fractures (**Figure 9.15a**).

Magnetic resonance imaging This is used to assess spinal cord injury (**Figure 9.15b**). STIR images can be used to identify symptomatic levels of marrow oedema to help decide which cases are suitable for vertebroplasty.

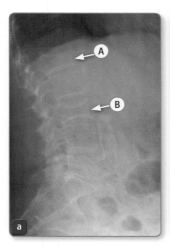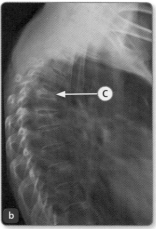

Figure 9.12 (a) Lateral radiograph of the lumbar spine, showing a grade 1 wedge fracture (A) of the L1 vertebra, as well as a grade 2 biconcave fracture (B) of the L3 vertebra. (b) Lateral radiograph of the thoracic spine, showing a grade 3 crush fracture (C) of the T5 vertebra.

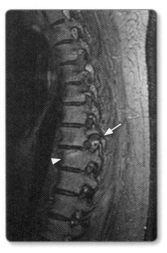

Figure 9.13 Sagittal short T1 inversion recovery magnetic resonance imaging, showing a T10 Chance fracture. A horizontal fracture line extends from the anterior vertebral body (arrowhead) to posterior elements (arrow).

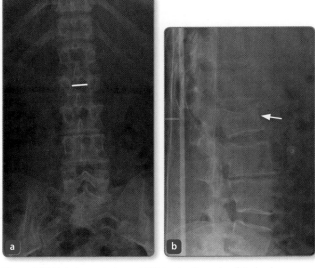

Figure 9.14 (a) Anteroposterior and (b) lateral radiographs of the lumbar spine, showing an L2 burst fracture (arrow). The interpedicular distance can be increased (white line) but is normal in this case.

Key imaging findings

- Vertebral body height is lost.
- Spinal alignment is lost.
- Widening of the paraspinal line indicates a haematoma.
- Transverse process fractures can be seen on the anteroposterior view (**Figure 9.16**).

Treatment

Stable fractures are treated conservatively with pain relief and spinal bracing. Unstable fractures may need spinal decompression and surgical fixation.

9.4 Facet injuries

Facet injuries are most commonly seen in cervical spine trauma.

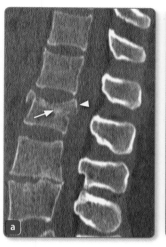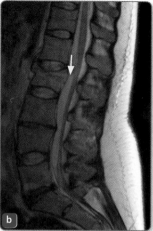

Figure 9.15 (a) Sagittal computerised tomography showing an L2 burst fracture (arrow) with posterior retropulsion (arrowhead) of the posterior portion. (b) Sagittal T1-weighted magnetic resonance imaging in the same patient showing no neurological compromise and good cerebrospinal fluid space anterior (arrow) to the cauda equina nerves.

Key facts

- Facet joints are bilateral. The right and left facet joints normally slightly overlap, but an abrupt change in overlap indicates rotational injury.
- The inferior articular facet should be in full contact with the superior articular facet of the vertebra below.
- Unilateral locked facet is caused by flexion injury, commonly occurring at C4–C5 and C5–C6.
- Bilateral locking of facets is also caused by flexion injury. It is strongly associated with spinal cord injury, due to the higher energy needed to dislocate both facets.

Radiological findings

Radiography Anteroposterior and lateral views are used to check alignment during the initial assessment of trauma.

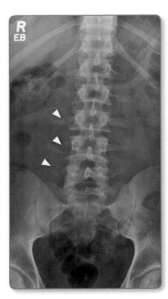

Figure 9.16 Anteroposterior radiograph of the lumbar spine, showing multiple right transverse process fractures at the right L3, L4 and L5 levels (arrow).

Computerised tomography The definitive investigation for assessing trauma is CT. CT of the cervical spine should extend from the skull base to T4 if facet injuries are suspected.

Key imaging finding
- Spinal alignment is lost.
  - Unilateral locked facet: there is loss of the normal straight line alignment of the spinous processes or vertebral bodies (**Figure 9.17**).
  - Bilateral locked facets: there is interruption of all spinal curves, total lack of facet joint articulation at the involved vertebral level, and horizontal displacement of a vertebral body by > 3.5 mm (**Figure 9.18**).

Treatment
Surgical fixation is usually needed. This may sometimes be done as an external fixation.

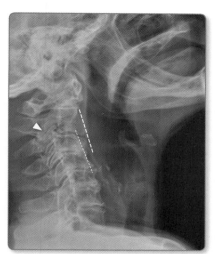

Figure 9.17 Lateral radiograph of the cervical spine, showing anterior subluxation of C2 vertebral alignment (thick dashed line) relative to C3 vertebral alignment (thin dashed line). This finding suggests locked unilateral facet, which was confirmed by the presence of overlapping of the facet (arrow).

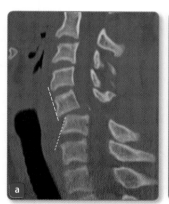
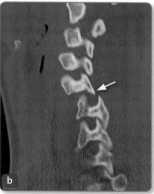

Figure 9.18 (a) Sagittal computerised tomography (CT) showing interruption of all spinal curves, including anterior vertebral alignment (thick and thin dashed lines). (b) Parasagittal CT confirmed the perched facets with complete lack of facet joint articulation (arrow).

9.5 Scoliosis

Scoliosis is lateral curvature of the spine in the coronal plane. Most cases are idiopathic, but scoliosis can also be congenital, developmental or neurological.

Key facts

- Scoliosis is classified by cause. Most cases (80%) are idiopathic.
  - Non-structural scoliosis can be postural or compensatory.
  - Transient structural scoliosis can be caused by sciatic pain or be psychosomatic or inflammatory.
  - Structural scoliosis can be idiopathic, congenital, neuromuscular or traumatic.
- Scoliosis also has a rotational component, accounting for the rib hump sometimes seen.

Radiological findings

Radiography Standing anteroposterior and lateral views are taken of the entire spine (**Figure 9.19**). The region of spine involved and which side of curvature is convex are important. Lateral bending views help when ascertaining whether the curvature corrects and the scoliosis is therefore non-structural.

Computerised tomography This is not typically needed except to assess congenital bony abnormalities, in which case the use of CT can help in surgical planning (**Figure 9.20**).

Magnetic resonance imaging To exclude an associated neurological pathology, MRI is frequently used.

Key imaging findings

- Cobb's angle is the maximal angle of the superior end plate of the uppermost vertebra to the inferior end plate of the lowermost vertebra involved in the curvature (**Figure 9.19**).
- The degree of rotation is estimated by the relation of the pedicles to the midline.
- With iliac crest apophyses, knowing the degree of ossification helps determine skeletal maturity.

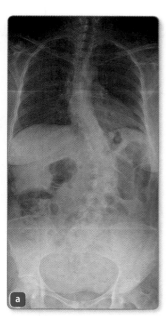

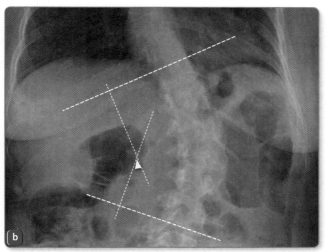

Figure 9.19 (a) Anteroposterior standing radiograph of the spine, showing scoliosis of the thoracolumbar spine, centred on L1 and convex to the left. (b) Close-up showing a Cobb's angle of 46° (arrowhead).

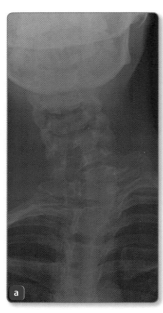

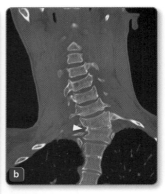

Figure 9.20 (a) Anteroposterior radiograph of the cervical spine, showing cervicothoracic scoliosis, convex to the left. (b) Sagittal computerised tomography confirmed congenital incomplete segmentation of T1 and T2 on the right side (arrowhead), with resultant congenital structural scoliosis.

Clinical insight

To find where the curvature starts and ends, look for the level with parallel end plates at its uppermost and lowermost portions. (thick dashed lines in Figure 9.19b). Perpendicular lines (thin dashed lines) are drawn from these thick dashed lines to obtain Cobb's angle

Treatment

Many cases of scoliosis can be treated conservatively. The decision whether or not to intervene operatively depends on the degree of curvature and the rate of growth expected, which in turn depends on the patient's age.

9.6 Spondylolisthesis

This is the spine (spondylo) slipping (listhesis), usually anterior displacement of a vertebra in relation to the vertebra below it. The commonest cause is spondylolytic (isthmic). Other causes are congenital (dysplastic), degenerative, traumatic and iatrogenic.

Key facts

- Spondylolytic spondylolisthesis results from defects in the pars interarticularis. Defects may be bilateral. It affects twice as many males as females.
- Typically, there is a combination of dysplastic pars at birth along with stresses from upright posture.
- Certain activities that extend the spine, such as diving, ballet or football (especially goalkeeping), increase these stresses.
- Degenerative spondylolisthesis is most frequent at the L4–L5 level. This type of spondylolisthesis is caused by the complex interaction of local structures rather than a pars defect.
- Retrolisthesis is the backward slippage of the vertebral body on the body below it. Retrolisthesis tends to be associated with facet joint osteoarthropathy.

Radiological findings

Radiography A lateral radiograph is used for visualising pars defects and for grading, which is slippage distance (**Figure 9.21a**) relative to vertebral body width (**Table 9.2**). Other features that may cause symptoms can also be assessed.

Computerised tomography Bony window images with sagittal reconstruction can confirm pars defect in suspected cases (**Figure 9.22**). Thin sections are useful for this purpose.

Nuclear medicine Increased activity on isotope bone scan can suggest spondylolisthesis, but the appearances are not specific.

Magnetic resonance imaging Paramedian sagittal images can show a fibrous bridge or pseudoarthrosis, both of which have sclerotic margins, seen as low signal intensity on all sequences. However, minimal sclerosis or similar signal intensity here can create false negatives on MRI. MRI also may show any potential spinal stenosis (**Figure 9.23**) or neuroforamina narrowing causing exiting nerve root entrapment (**Figure 9.21c**).

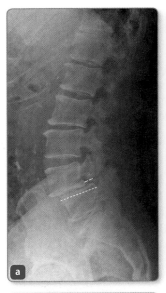

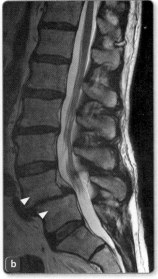

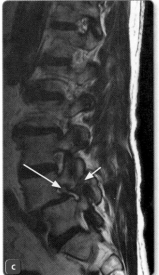

Figure 9.21 (a) Lateral radiograph of the lumbar spine, showing grade 2 spondylolisthesis of L4 on L5. The amount of slip (thick dashed line) is 25–49% of the total vertebral width (thin dashed line). (b) Sagittal magnetic resonance imaging (MRI) of the lumbar spine, showing type 2 Modic changes (arrowheads) in adjacent L4–L5 end plates. (c) Right parasagittal MRI showing a pars defect (short arrow) causing severe right neuroforamina narrowing (long arrow) with resultant impingement of the exiting right L4 nerve root.

Grade	Slip relative to vertebral anteroposterior width (%)
1	0 to < 25
2	25 to < 50
3	50 to < 75
4	75–100

Table 9.2 Grading of spondylolisthesis

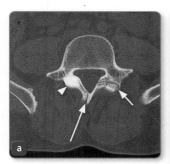

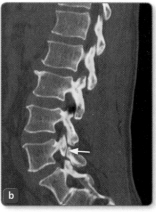

Figure 9.22 (a) Axial and (b) parasagittal computerised tomography of the lumbar spine, showing a unilateral pars defect on the left side (short arrows). On the right side is an expanded sclerosis of the pars (arrowhead). The unfused spinous process (long arrow) is an incidental finding consistent with spina bifida occulta.

Key imaging finding

- Oblique lumbar spine views (**Figure 9.24**) demonstrate a 'Scottie dog with collar' appearance due to pars defect. This can be observed on oblique reconstructions from multislice CT scanning

Treatment

Treatment depends on factors such as age, extent of slip and severity of symptoms. Treatment of most cases of spondylolisthesis is conservative and includes rest and epidural injections. Surgery is reserved for cases in which conservative treatment

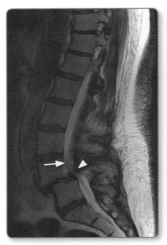

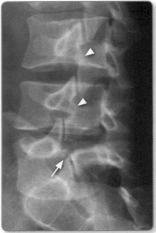

Figure 9.23 Sagittal T2-weighted magnetic resonance imaging of the lumbar spine, showing grade 2 spondylolisthesis of L4 on L5, resulting in spinal stenosis (arrowhead). The cauda equina nerve roots are bunched up proximal to the stenosis (arrow).

Figure 9.24 Oblique radiograph of the lumbar spine, showing the pars defect (arrow). The defect forms the collar on what looks like a Scottie dog on the L5 vertebra. Compare with the normal intact pars interarticularis at the levels above (arrowheads).

fails and usually consists of decompression, spinal fusion or both.

9.7 Intervertebral disc herniation

Intervertebral discs contain nucleus pulposus centrally, bounded by annulus fibrosis.

Key facts

- More than a third of asymptomatic adults have a detectable disc herniation.
- Sciatica is the radicular pain that occurs when a nerve root is impinged on by the herniated disc (or other pathology).

- It is important to distinguish radicular pain, which is dermatomal, from referred pain, which is non-dermatomal.

Radiological findings

Radiography This imaging modality can visualise only indirect features of reduced intervertebral disc height. Herniation cannot be visualised by plain radiographs.

Computerised tomography This is used when MRI is contraindicated. CT is also useful to show bony canal narrowing by syndesmophytes. CT myelography can be done in some cases when there is discrepancy between clinical symptoms and MRI findings.

Magnetic resonance imaging The modality of choice for intervertebral disc herniation is MRI. The position of the disc material is described precisely (**Figure 9.25**). Herniation of the nucleus pulposus into the spinal canal causes the annulus fibrosus to protrude posteriorly. Disc tissue extending cranially or caudally beyond the vertebral end plates is considered an extrusion (**Figure 9.26a**) instead of a protrusion. If the disc fragment becomes separated, this is a sequestered disc (**Figure 9.26b**).

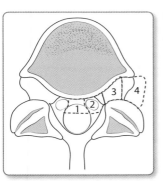

Figure 9.25 The central (1), paracentral or subarticular (2), foraminal (3) and extraforaminal or far lateral (4) sites of disc herniation.

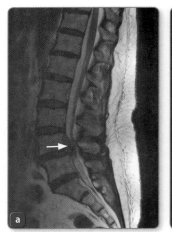 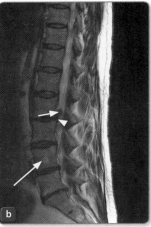

Figure 9.26 Sagittal T2-weighted magnetic resonance imaging of the lumbar spine. (a) An extruded L4–L5 disc with herniation extending cranially (arrow). (b) A sequestered fragment (short arrow) separated from L2–L3 disc herniation (arrowhead). At the L4 vertebral body is an incidental haemangioma (long arrow).

- Paracentral disc herniation (**Figure 9.27**) occupies the lateral recess and impinges on the transiting nerve root (e.g. L5 at the L4–L5 level)
- **Foraminal disc herniation** (**Figure 9.28**) or stenosis causes impingement of the exiting nerve root (e.g. L4 at the L4 level)
- **Large disc herniation** can cause spinal stenosis or cauda equina syndrome (see section 9.9, Spinal stenosis and cord compression)

Key imaging findings
- End plate Modic changes may be relevant (see **Table 9.3**).
- With an annular tear, look for focal or linear hyperintensity in a hypointense annulus fibrosis on T2-weighted MRI (**Figure 9.29**).
- Post-surgery scar tissue can be distinguished from recurrent disc disease by contrast enhancement (**Figure 9.30**).

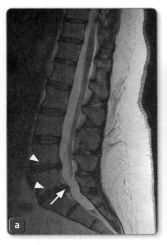
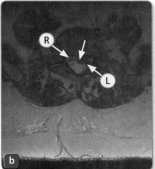

Figure 9.27 (a) Sagittal and (b) axial T2-weighted magnetic resonance imaging of the lumbar spine, showing L5–S1 left paracentral disc herniation (short arrows) causing encroachment of the left lateral recess and displacing the transiting left S1 nerve root ((L)). The right S1 nerve root (R) remains normal. Note the type 2 Modic changes (arrowheads) adjacent to L4–L5 and L5–S1.

Treatment

Spontaneous resolution of disc herniation occurs in over a third of cases. Failed conservative treatment may necessitate discectomy.

9.8 Discitis

Discitis is infection of the intervertebral disc space. In spondylodiscitis, the vertebral end plates are involved. Most infections are of haematogenous origin. Predisposing immunocompromised states and previous local surgery are risk factors.

Key facts

- In pyogenic discitis, the commonest organism is *Staphylococcus aureus*. *Streptococcus* is more frequent in endocarditis. *Pseudomonas aeruginosa* is common in intravenous drug users.

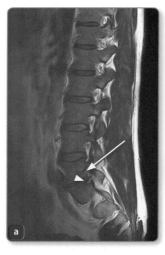

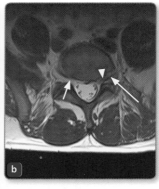

Figure 9.28 Left (a) parasagittal and (b) axial T2-weighted magnetic resonance imaging of the lumbar spine, showing L5–S1 left foraminal disc herniation (arrowheads) causing stenosis of the left neural foramina and impinging on the exiting left L5 nerve root (long arrows). Contrast with the normal right neural foramina (short arrow).

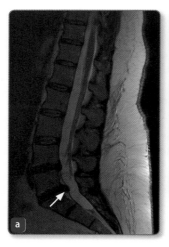

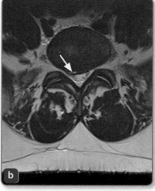

Figure 9.29 (a) Sagittal and (b) axial T2-weighted magnetic resonance imaging of the lumbar spine, showing the high-signal periphery (arrow) of L5–S1 right paracentral disc herniation, consistent with an annular tear.

Type	T1-weighted	T2-weighted	Pathological change
1	Hypointense	Hyperintense	Oedema
2	Hyperintense	Hyperintense	Fatty change
3	Hypointense	Hypointense	Sclerosis
[a] Mixed types can be present. Type 3 changes are rare.			

Table 9.3 Signal changes on magnetic resonance imaging associated with different Modic types[a]

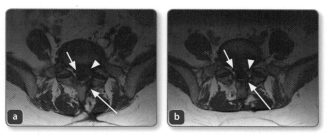

Figure 9.30 Axial (a) precontrast and (b) post-contrast T1-weighted magnetic resonance imaging of the lumbar spine at the L5–S1 level, showing a low-signal lesion (arrowhead) at the left lateral recess in part (a). In the post-contrast view (b), a rim of enhancing scar tissue encases the transiting left S1 nerve root (arrowhead). The right S1 nerve root (short arrows) remains normal. Note the previous left laminectomy (long arrows).

- Chronic discitis typically has an indolent presentation. *Mycobacterium tuberculosis* (which causes tuberculosis) is the commonest organism, in which case the condition is known as Pott's disease. The disease is usually related to immunodeficiency states.
- The involvement of posterior elements may lead to collapse and neurological complications. Healed disease can result in fusion and kyphoscoliosis.

Radiological findings

Radiography Irregular end plates and loss of disc height may take a few weeks to become apparent (**Figure 9.31**).

In spondylodiscitis, osteopaenia is evident only after over half the vertebral body has been destroyed. Chronic disease can lead to vertebral destruction and consequent kyphosis; some cases show vertebral fusion.

Computerised tomography Other than showing the end plates and vertebral body destruction (**Figure 9.32**), CT can visualise associated paravertebral abscesses.

Nuclear medicine Technetium or gallium scans are positive but non-specific. Gallium scans become negative after treatment, whereas technetium scans may remain positive.

Magnetic resonance imaging This is the imaging modality of choice in suspected discitis and for follow-up. MRI is the best method for early detection.

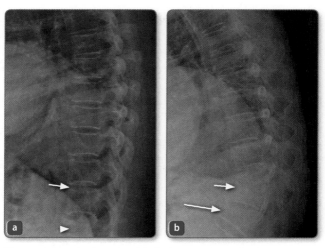

Figure 9.31 Lateral radiographs of the lumbar spine. (a) Initial radiograph taken for an acute wedge fracture of the L1 vertebra (arrowhead) The T11/12 disc space appears normal at this stage (arrow). (b) Radiograph taken 3 months later, showing the healed fracture (long arrow) but collapsed T11–T12 anteriorly, with loss of end plate definition and disc height (short arrow). The kyphosis has increased as a result.

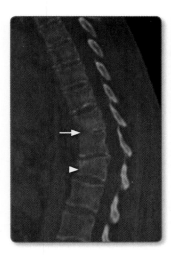

Figure 9.32 Sagittal computerised tomography of the thoracolumbar spine (same patient as Figure 9.31), showing reduced disc height, bony destruction and irregular end plate margins anteriorly at T11–T12 (arrow). The patient had an established history of L1 anterior wedge fracture (arrowhead).

Early discitis shows atypical signal characteristics, and the end plates may be initially spared. There is low signal on T1-weighted and high signal on T2-weighted MRI at the infected disc and adjacent end plates (**Figure 9.33**). Also visible is an associated abnormal marrow signal, consistent with oedema and infiltration. Gadolinium contrast shows variable enhancement, which can be homogeneous or heterogeneous, and complete or peripheral involvement. Focal vertebral body osteolysis and abscesses show rim enhancement.

Key imaging findings

- Radiographs show initial loss of definition of the end plates and decrease in disc space height. Next is vertebral body lucency with loss of trabeculations. Last, frank bone destruction is visible.
- There is reduced disc space with irregular end plates.
- Prevertebral and epidural abscesses are visible (**Figure 9.34**).

Clinical insight

In children, whose higher red marrow content gives low to intermediate background signal, discitis showing as low signal on T1-weighted MRI can be more difficult to diagnose.

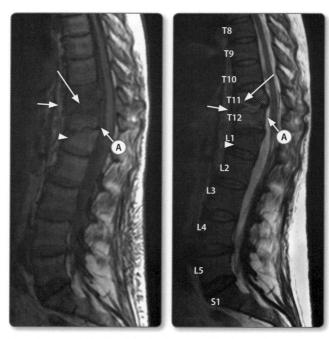

Figure 9.33 Sagittal (a) T1-weighted and (b) T2-weighted magnetic resonance imaging of the lumbar spine, showing discitis at T11–T12, with low-signal T1-weighted and high-signal T2-weighted end plates (long arrow) and loss of disc space. A prevertebral abscess is visible anteriorly (short arrows) and an epidural abscess posteriorly Ⓐ in the spinal canal. An established old L1 grade I anterior wedge fracture is present (arrowheads).

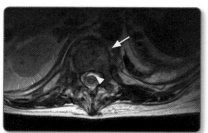

Figure 9.34 Axial T2-weighted magnetic resonance imaging of the lumbar spine, showing a prevertebral abscess on the left (arrow) and an epidural abscess (arrowhead) anterior to the spinal cord.

Treatment

A course of intravenous antibiotics for 6–12 weeks is usually needed. Cases that are resistant to treatment, or that involve significant abscesses or the development of neurological complications, may need surgical intervention. Surgery often involves spinal stabilisation.

9.9 Spinal stenosis and cord compression

Spinal stenosis is narrowing of the spinal canal (**Figure 9.35**). Acute spinal stenosis at the level of the spinal cord may cause cord compression. If this occurs at the level of the cauda equina, cauda equina syndrome may result (**Figure 9.36**). More often, chronic cervical or lumbar stenosis occurs gradually, typically because of a combination of degenerative disc, facet and ligamentum hypertrophy (**Figures 9.38** to **9.40**). Tumours and spinal injuries may also be a cause.

Key facts

- Congenital spinal stenosis (**Figure 9.35**) is often asymptomatic until late adulthood.

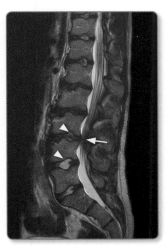

Figure 9.35 Sagittal T2-weighted magnetic resonance imaging of the lumbar spine, showing congenital spinal stenosis at L3–L4 (arrow). The biconcave internal disc herniations are consistent with multiple levels of Schmorl's node formation (arrowheads).

- Cervical stenosis may present with myelopathy (subtle loss of hand dexterity, hyper-reflexia and mild proximal lower limb weakness).
- Lumbar stenosis presents with neurogenic claudication. Neurogenic claudication, unlike vascular claudication, is unrelieved by rest. Features include bilateral leg pain, which worsens with walking and prolonged standing and is relieved by changing position or lumbar flexion.

Clinical insight

Cauda equina syndrome occurs when a large acutely herniated disc compresses the entire spinal canal and the cauda equina nerve roots are compressed (**Figure 9.36**). Patients present with bilateral leg pain; urinary, rectal or sexual dysfunction; and so-called saddle paraesthesia.

Cauda equina syndrome is a clinical emergency and urgent MRI is indicated. Early surgery may prevent long-term neurological sequelae.

Radiological findings

Radiography Radiography is not useful, except to rule out other causes of back pain.

Computerised tomography This is used for patients for whom MRI is contra-indicated. CT is also used

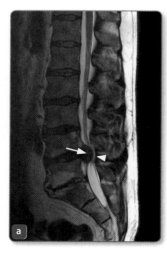

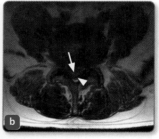

Figure 9.36 (a) Sagittal and (b) axial T2-weighted magnetic resonance imaging of the lumbar spine, showing acute large L4–L5 central disc herniation (arrows). This causes compression of the dural sac (arrowheads) and the presentation of cauda equina syndrome.

to assess bony or calcified structures to help surgical planning.

Magnetic resonance imaging This is the investigation of choice for spinal stenosis and cord compression. A narrowed spinal canal with reduced dural sac volume is visible (**Figure 9.37**). Chronic cord compression may result in myelomalacia (**Figure 9.38**). Other pathologies, such as tumour

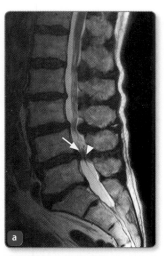

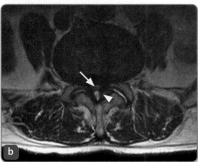

Figure 9.37 (a) Sagittal and (b) axial T2-weighted magnetic resonance imaging of the lumbar spine, showing lumbar spinal stenosis at L4–L5 caused by a combination of disc, ligamentum and facet hypertrophy, which is worse on the left (arrowheads). These views show the narrowed spinal canal (arrow) with bunched-up proximal cauda equina.

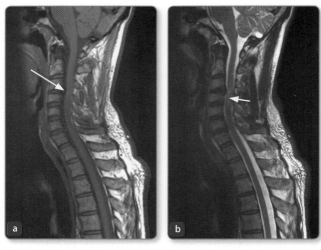

Figure 9.38 Sagittal (a) T1-weighted and (b) T2-weighted magnetic resonance imaging of the cervical spine, showing C3–C4 disc herniation (long arrow) causing cervical spinal stenosis. The long-standing increased signal changes in the spinal cord (short arrow) are consistent with myelomalacia.

(**Figure 9.39**) or synovial cyst (**Figure 9.40**) from degenerative facet joint, can cause spinal stenosis.

Key imaging findings

- Look for compression of the spinal cord or cauda equina nerves in the dural sac.
- There is loss of cerebrospinal fluid anterior and posterior to the cord or cauda equina nerves.
- Myelomalacia with increased fluid signal is present in chronic cord compression.

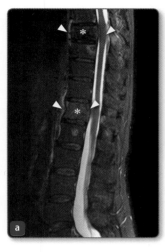

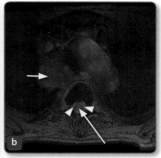

Figure 9.39 Magnetic resonance imaging (MRI) of the thoracolumbar spine. (a) Sagittal short T1 inversion recovery MRI showing soft tissue extension (arrowheads) of thoracic metastatic disease at T8 and T12 (*) encasing the spinal cord at the T8 level, with early features at T12. There is also anterior prevertebral tumour extension. (b) Axial T2-weighted MRI showing the tumour (arrowheads) encasing the spinal cord (long arrow). In the lung a hilar mass is present (arrow).

- Bunching up of cauda equina nerves proximal to stenosis is visible on the sagittal view.

Treatment

Management depends on the presentation and cause. Acute presentations of cord compression or cauda equina syndrome may need urgent decompression. Decompression can also be used in some chronic cases. Radiotherapy may be suitable for patients with tumours causing stenosis.

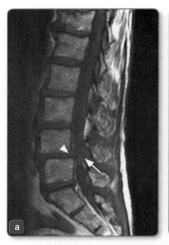

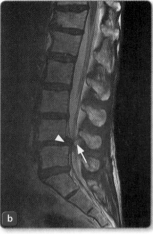

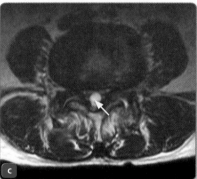

Figure 9.40 Sagittal (a) T1-weighted and (b) T2-weighted magnetic resonance imaging (MRI) of the lumbar spine, showing grade 1 spondylolisthesis of L4 on L5 with mild broad-based disc herniation (arrowheads). A lesion is present posteriorly, showing low signal on T1 weighting and high signal on T2 weighting, consistent with a facet joint synovial cyst. (c) Axial T2-weighted MRI confirms the synovial cyst (short arrows) causing spinal stenosis.

Bony lesions

chapter 10

10.1 Bone tumours

Most bone tumours are benign. Malignant bone tumours are usually caused by metastatic disease. Primary malignant bone tumours are rare. It is more useful to characterise bony lesions as aggressive or non-aggressive rather than malignant or benign, respectively (**Figure 10.1**), because some malignant lesions grow slowly and some benign lesions, such as acute osteomyelitis, can seem aggressive.

When characterising a bony lesion, consider the following factors.

- The patient's age: broadly, differential diagnosis depends on whether the patient is younger or older than 30 years. However, some lesions, such as those caused by infection, can occur at any age (see **Figure 10.2**).

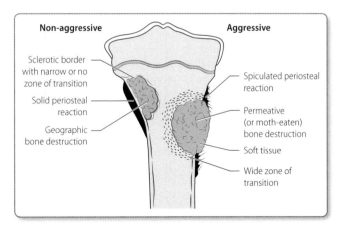

Figure 10.1 The different characteristics of non-aggressive and aggressive bony lesions.

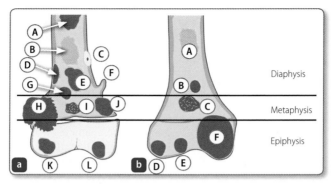

Figure 10.2 Types and sites of bony tumours by patient age. (a) Bony tumours in patients aged < 30 years. (A) Fibrous dysplasia, (B) Ewing's eosinophilic granuloma, (C) osteoid osteoma, (D) non-ossifying fibroma, (E) simple bone cyst, (F) osteochondroma, (G) chondromyxoid fibroma, (H) osteosarcoma, (I) enchondroma, (J) aneurysmal bone cyst, (K) chondroblastoma, (L) infection. (a) Bony tumours in patients aged > 30 years. (A) Metastasis, myeloma or lymphoma; (B) metastasis, myeloma or Brown tumour of hyperparathyroidism; (C) enchondroma or chondrosarcoma; (D) geode; (E) infection; (F) giant cell tumour.

- The morphological characteristics of the lesion: what the lesion looks like and whether or not bone destruction or formation is present. If the lesion is destructive, consider the pattern of destruction. The characteristics of the zone of transition, that is, the edge of the lesion, also help decide whether or not the lesion is aggressive (see **Table 10.1**).
- The site of the lesion: different tumours are commoner in different sites of the body, such as the axial skeleton or certain long bones. Different bony tumours tend to be found in the epiphysis (only a few types of lesion), the metaphysis or the diaphysis (**Figure 10.2**). In the long bones, most tumours are eccentric (i.e. non-central). Medullary (central) tumours include simple bone cysts, enchondroma, eosinophilic granuloma and fibrous dysplasia.
- Periosteal reaction: different patterns of periosteal reaction may provide information about the lesion (**Figure 10.3**).

Morphological characteristics of bony lesion	Non-aggressive bone tumour	Aggressive bone tumour
Type of lesion	Sclerotic (white)	Lytic (lucent)
Pattern of destruction	Geographic pattern (well-circumscribed, possibly with a sclerotic rim)	Two possible patterns: • moth-eaten pattern (numerous poorly circumscribed lesions) • permeative pattern (widespread elongated perforations along the bone cortex)
Zone of transition	Well-defined, with a narrow zone of transition	Ill-defined, with a wide zone of transition

Table 10.1 Morphological characteristics of non-aggressive and aggressive bone tumours

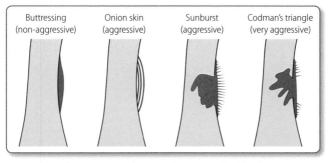

Buttressing (non-aggressive)   Onion skin (aggressive)   Sunburst (aggressive)   Codman's triangle (very aggressive)

Figure 10.3 Different patterns of periosteal reaction ordered by degree of aggressiveness.

A single thick layer of periosteal reaction can form a buttress. This finding is non-specific but usually indicates a slow-growing, non-aggressive lesion. The lamellated onion skin pattern of periosteal reaction is consistent with an aggressive lesion. The sunburst or hair-on-end pattern produces numerous spicules arising from the centre of an aggressive lesion. Codman's triangle is formed by periosteal elevation at the edge of a tumour and indicates a very aggressive lesion.

- Tumour matrix: tumours can be one of three types (osteoid, chondroid or fibrous), depending on the tumour matrix they produce (**Table 10.2**). Osteoid, chondroid and fibrous tumours have benign and malignant forms.
- Soft tissue expansion: aggressive lesions often have soft tissue invasion with resultant soft tissue swelling. These features are visible as increased adjacent density on radiography.

Key facts

- In older patients, always consider metastases, multiple myeloma or lymphoma.
- Tumours of the bronchus, breast, prostate and kidney can metastasise to bone.
- Solitary bone cysts, aneurysmal bone cysts, histiocytosis, fibrous dysplasia, Brown tumour of hyperparathyroidism and myositis ossificans can mimic bone tumour.

Nature of tumour	Osteoid[*]	Chondroid[†]	Fibrous[‡]
Benign	• Osteoid osteoma • Osteoblastoma • Osteoma • Enostosis (bone island)	• Enchondroma • Osteochondroma • Chondroblastoma • Chondromyxoid fibroma	• Fibrous cortical defect • Non-ossifying fibroma
Malignant	• Osteosarcoma	• Chondrosarcoma	• Fibrosarcoma • Malignant fibrous histiocytoma

*Bone forming: fluffy cloud or cotton-like densities visible in lesion.
†Cartilage forming: so-called popcorn, comma-shaped or annular calcifications visible.
‡Fibrous forming: homogenous, lucent lesions.

Table 10.2 Different matrix-forming bone tumours

Radiological findings

Radiography The most helpful investigation for bone tumours is a radiograph. Morphological characteristics, the site of the lesion and the type of local reaction all help to determine the aggressiveness of the tumour and rule out differential diagnoses.

Ultrasound This modality is of limited use for diagnosis. However, ultrasound can be used to assess the soft tissue element. Ultrasound is also used for imaging-guided biopsy.

Computerised tomography This is useful for osseous assessment. Computerised tomography (CT) can also be used to detect pulmonary metastases as a staging examination.

Bone scan The results of a bone scan can help surgical planning by determining if a lesion is solitary or multifocal. Indeterminate lesions can be checked for metabolic activity.

Magnetic resonance imaging This modality is excellent for assessing tumour extent, that is, local staging. Magnetic resonance imaging (MRI) is usually combined with fat-suppressed, contrast-enhanced sequences. It is used to determine the exact margins of the lesion to help in surgical planning.

Key imaging findings
- When assessing the morphological characteristics of a lesion, note the pattern of destruction and the zone of transition.
- Note the site of the lesion: the region of the bone (medullary or eccentric) and the region of the body.
- Note whether the periosteal reaction has non-aggressive or aggressive features.
- Examine the tumour matrix for the presence of bony, cartilaginous or fibrous tissue.
- Soft tissue swelling indicates an aggressive lesion.

Treatment
Treatment depends on the histological characteristics of the lesion. Treatment is usually surgical, ranging from wide local excision to radical resection.

Benign bone tumours

Simple bone cyst

Simple bone cysts appear in the first 20 years of life and are three times more common in males. The cysts are asymptomatic but may present as a pathological fracture.

Simple bone cysts are found in the metaphysis of a long bone, abutting the growth plate. They can be central or intra-medullary and may expand the bone.

On radiography, simple bone cysts are visible as well-defined lucencies with no periosteal reaction. They are sometimes multiloculated. Look for the fallen fragment sign, that is, the presence of a bone fragment in the lesion (**Figure 10.4**).

Aneurysmal bone cyst

Most aneurysmal bone cysts are found in people younger than 20 years and may present with pain. The name is a misnomer, because an aneurysmal bone cyst is neither an aneurysm nor a cyst. It is an arteriovenous fistula in a bone.

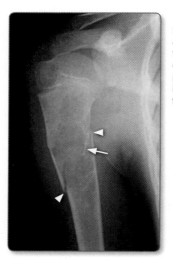

Figure 10.4 Anteroposterior radiograph of the right shoulder of an adolescent with a pathological fracture (arrowheads). The fracture was caused by a simple bone cyst of the proximal humerus. A bone fragment is visible (arrow); this is the fallen fragment sign.

Aneurysmal bone cysts are located eccentrically in the metaphysis of long bones and the spine. The cyst is a well-defined expansile osteolytic lesion with thin sclerotic margins (**Figure 10.5a**). Fluid–fluid levels are visible on CT or MRI (**Figure 10.5b,c**).

Fibrous cortical defect and non-ossifying fibroma

Fibrous cortical defects and non-ossifying fibromas are found in children aged 2–15 years. They are twice as common in boys and are one of the most common benign lesions.

These bone tumours occur in the distal femur or in the proximal or distal tibia. On radiographs, the tumour is visible as a lucency with a thin sclerotic rim (**Figure 10.6a,b**). The rest of the lesion may heal spontaneously and disappear or it may become sclerotic as it heals in adulthood (**Figure 10.6c**).

Osteoid osteoma

Most osteoid osteomas are found in patients aged 10–35 years. They are two to four times more common in males. The tumours cause night pain that is relieved by aspirin. If the spine is involved, patients may experience painful scoliosis.

Osteoid osteomas are found in long bones, phalanges and vertebrae. They may appear normal. Alternatively, they may show diffuse periosteal reaction with cortical thickening and a well-circumscribed lucent nidus with a central sclerotic dot, best seen on CT (**Figure 10.7**). MRI shows non-specific marrow oedema. On isotope bone scan, look for the double-density sign: a central intense focus surrounded by a rim of less intense but increased uptake.

Enchondroma

Enchondromas occur between the ages of 10 and 30 years. The tumour is usually asymptomatic but may cause a pathological fracture. Malignant transformation is rare.

Chondrosarcomas may arise from multiple enchondromas in Ollier's disease or Maffucci's syndrome (with additional multiple haemangiomas). These tumours are found in the small tubular

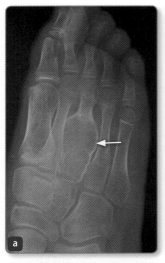

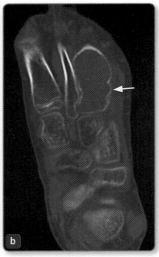

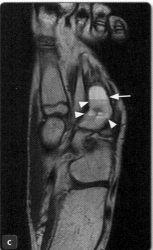

Figure 10.5 (a) Oblique radiograph of the left foot, showing a well-defined expansile lucent lesion with thin sclerotic margins (arrow) in the 3rd metacarpal metaphysis. (b) The lesion is outlined (arrow) on computerised tomography coronal reconstruction. (b) Multiple fluid–fluid levels (arrowheads) in the lesion (arrow) are visible on coronal T2-weighted magnetic resonance imaging.

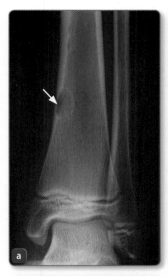
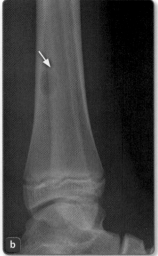
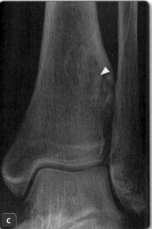

Figure 10.6 (a) Anterior and (b) lateral radiographs of the left ankle, showing a well-defined eccentric metaphyseal lesion with a thin rim (arrows), consistent with a fibrous cortical defect. (c) The lesion calcifies (arrowhead) in adulthood.

bones of the hands and feet or in large long bones. They have a medullary (i.e. central) location.

Look for small lytic lesions with a narrow zone of transition and sharp endosteal scalloping. Expansion may be present without a cortical break, unless the bone is fractured (**Figure 10.8**). Chondroid calcification may be visible as rings and arcs.

Osteochondroma

Osteochondromas develop in childhood but persist into adulthood. They present as incidental findings or through the effects

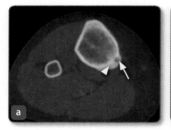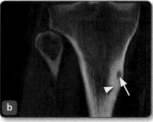

Figure 10.7 (a) Axial and (b) coronal computerised tomography reconstructions of the right tibia, showing a well-defined lucency representing the nidus (arrows) of an osteoid osteoma. Cortical thickening (arrowheads) surrounds the lesion. No central sclerotic dot is visible in the nidus in this example.

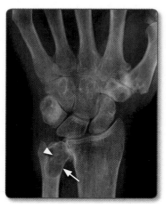

Figure 10.8 Anteroposterior radiograph of the left wrist, showing a well-defined expansile lucent lesion with sharp endosteal scalloping (arrow). These findings are consistent with enchondroma. Chondroid calcification (arrowhead) is present.

of impingement of nearby tissue. Multiple osteochondromas occur in hereditary multiple exostoses (diaphyseal aclasis).

Osteochondromas are appendicular, especially around the knee. They are metaphyseal, projecting away from the epiphysis (**Figure 10.9a**), and can be sessile or pedunculated.

New growth after maturity or any aggressive features are typical of malignant transformation, which occurs in 1% of solitary osteochondromas and 5% of multiple osteochondromas. Use MRI to assess the thickness of the cartilage cap of the osteochondroma, which may be thin or thick with chondroid calcification (**Figure 10.9b**). A cartilage cap > 1.5 cm thick suggests malignant change.

Fibrous dysplasia

Three quarters of patients with fibrous dysplasia present at less than 30 years of age. If fibrous dysplasia is associated with endocrinopathy, it is known as McCune–Albright syndrome. If it is associate with soft tissue myxomas, it is called Mazabraud's syndrome.

Fibrous dysplasia is the progressive painless replacement of normal bone with immature woven bone. The condition may

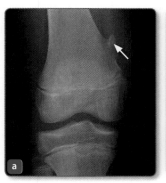 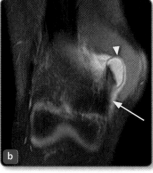

Figure 10.9 (a) Anteroposterior radiograph of the right knee, showing a pedunculated osteochondroma (arrow), projecting away from the epiphysis. (b) Coronal short T1 inversion recovery magnetic resonance imaging shows the cartilage cap (arrowhead) with mild adjacent soft tissue fluid (long arrow) caused by soft tissue irritation.

be mono-ostic, involving a single bone, or polyostic, involving multiple bones. It can be craniofacial, affecting the skull and facial bones only, or it can affect the mandible and maxilla only (causing cherubism).

Almost any bone may be affected. The ribs are most commonly involved in mono-ostic cases. The lesion is well circumscribed, with ground glass opacities. Its appearance may be mixed, or it may be completely lucent or sclerotic. The bone is expanded (**Figure 10.10**). Fibrous dysplasia may appear aggressive on MRI and is metabolically active on isotope bone scan.

Giant cell tumour

Giant cell tumours occur mostly after closure of the growth plates, typically between the ages of 20 and 30 years. They may present as bone pain, soft tissue mass, local compression

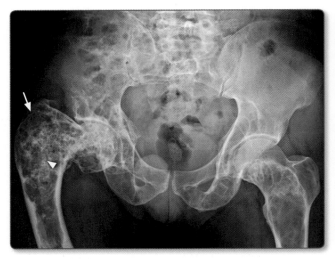

Figure 10.10 Anteroposterior radiograph of the pelvis, showing a polyostotic form of fibrous dysplasia. The proximal femora and pelvis are affected bilaterally but more extensively on the right. The ground glass appearance (arrowhead) and gross expansion of the bones (arrow) are characteristic.

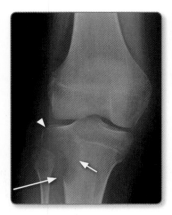

Figure 10.11 Anteroposterior radiograph of the right knee, showing a giant cell tumour. The well-defined lucent lesion with a non-sclerotic margin (short arrow) shows expansile features (long arrow) and extends to the articular surface (arrowhead).

or pathological fractures. Between 5 to 10% of these lesions are malignant.

The commonest presentation is a singular lesion around the knee (**Figure 10.11**). Distal radius and sacral lesions are also possible. Multiple lesions are present in only 1% of cases.

Giant cell tumours appear as lucent, eccentric lesions with a well-defined non-sclerotic margin abutting the articular surface. Some cases involve periosteal reactions. In contrast to aneurysmal bone cysts, enhancing solid components are visible on MRI. On bone scan, look for a doughnut sign with central photopaenia.

Malignant bone tumours
Ewing's sarcoma

Ewing's sarcoma usually presents between the ages of 10 and 20 years. They experience non-specific localised pain. A soft tissue mass may be present.

Long bones, usually the femur, are affected in 60% of cases. Flat bones, usually the pelvis and scapula (**Figure 10.12**), are affected in 40% of cases. Ewing's sarcoma is typically diaphyseal. Aggressive features include a permeative pattern, a laminated periosteal reaction and sclerosis in some cases.

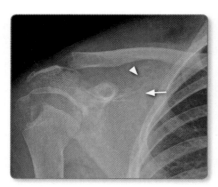

Figure 10.12
Anteroposterior radiograph of the right shoulder, showing the permeative bony destruction (arrow) of Ewing's sarcoma, with laminated periosteal reaction (arrowhead).

Osteosarcoma

Three quarters of patients presenting with osteosarcoma at less than than 20 years of age have primary osteosarcoma. In elderly patients it is secondary to malignant degeneration of Paget's disease (see section 10.3), extensive bony infarcts or radiotherapy. Osteosarcoma usually presents with bone pain and soft tissue swelling.

Osteosarcoma is found in the metadiaphysis of long bones, typically around the knee (**Figure 10.13**). The innominate, maxilla and mandible, or vertebrae can also be affected. Look for medullary and cortical bone destruction with a permeative or moth-eaten pattern, as well as a wide zone of transition. The periosteal reaction, a sunburst pattern or Codman's triangle, is aggressive. The tumour matrix is variable: fluffy or cloud-like. Use MRI to evaluate soft tissue involvement for local staging.

Chondrosarcoma

Chondrosarcoma usually presents at the age of 30–50 years. The tumour causes pain, pathological fracture or a lump.

Chondrosarcomas are found in long bones such as the distal femur, the proximal tibia and the proximal humerus. They can also occur in the pelvis, ribs and spine. Half of these tumours are lytic, and most have calcifications (chondroid or popcorn). Higher grade chondrosarcomas can appear moth-eaten or

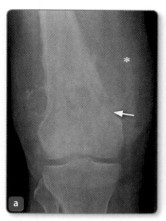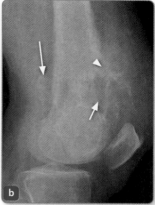

Figure 10.13 (a) Anteroposterior and (b) lateral radiographs of the right knee, showing an osteosarcoma at the distal femoral metaphysis. Medullary and cortical bony destruction (short arrows) with extension of the tumour has caused Codman's triangle (arrowhead) and sunburst (long arrow) periosteal reactions. Extensive soft tissue swelling is present (*).

permeative. Endosteal scalloping is more extensive than in enchondroma. Cortical remodelling and periosteal reaction are present.

Metastatic lesions

Skeletal metastases account for 70% of bone tumours. Most are asymptomatic, but patients occasionally present with local bone pain, soft tissue mass complications or pathological fractures.

Metastatic lesions are found in the vertebrae (especially the posterior vertebral body, extending into the pedicles), the pelvis, the proximal femur and humerus and the skull. Lesions may appear lytic, sclerotic (typically prostate cancer in men and breast cancers in women) or mixed sclerotic and lytic (**Figure 10.14a**).

Isotope bone scanning is a very sensitive modality for identifying diffuse metastatic disease (**Figure 10.14b**). CT can

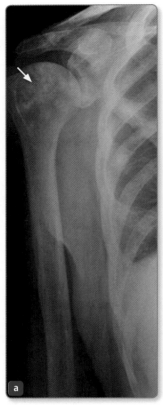

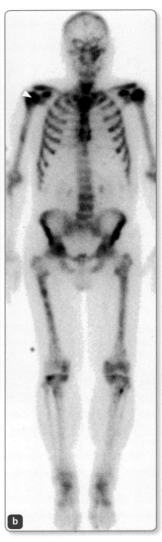

Figure 10.14 (a) Anteroposterior radiograph confirming sclerotic metastases (arrow) in the right proximal humerus. (b) Anterior whole-body isotope bone scan demonstrating increased uptake in the right proximal humerus (arrowhead). There are widespread metabolically active multiple bony metastases.

determine bony involvement and risk of pathological fractures. MRI is highly sensitive for identifying marrow replacement.

Multiple myeloma

Multiple myeloma is the commonest primary bone malignancy in adults. It is usually disseminated, with multiple defined lesions or diffuse skeletal osteopaenia. Solitary plasmacytoma is a single large expansile lesion, usually in a vertebral body or the pelvis. Osteosclerotic myeloma is rare. These tumours present with bone pain, anaemia, renal failure or hypercalcaemia. The patient may have pathological fractures.

Multiple myeloma mostly affects the axial skeleton (usually the vertebrae) and proximal appendicular bones. A skeletal survey shows purely lytic, sharply defined or punched-out lesions with endosteal scalloping (**Figure 10.15**). Marrow infiltration is exquisitely visualised on MRI. The isotope bone scan may be negative because of a lack of osteoblastic activity.

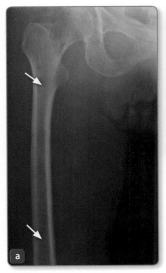

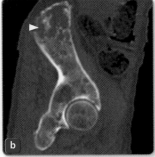

Figure 10.15 (a) Anteroposterior radiograph of the right femur, showing multiple small lucencies without sclerotic edges throughout the entire bone (arrows), consistent with multiple myeloma. (b) Sagittal computerised tomography showing further lesions in the pelvis (arrowhead).

Lymphoma

Lymphoma is a rare primary condition in the bones. It may present with pain or mass, along with systemic B symptoms (fever, night sweats and weight loss). Secondary involvement of the bone marrow is common in systemic lymphoma.

Lymphoma can affect any part of the skeleton, but is most commonly found in the spine and long bones. The tumour has a variable appearance, ranging from normal to lytic, blastic or both lytic and blastic. A periosteal reaction may be present (**Figure 10.16a**). MRI is essential to show bone marrow replacement as well as soft tissue involvement (**Figure 10.16b**).

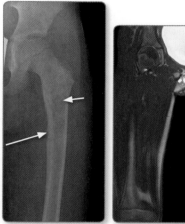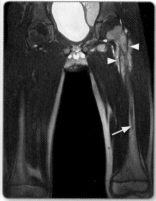

Figure 10.16 (a) Anteroposterior radiograph of the left femur, showing an ill-defined area of lucency with a wide zone of transition (short arrow). Periosteal changes are visible (long arrow). (b) Coronal T2-weighted magnetic resonance imaging showing widespread marrow replacement by lymphoma, with an altered signal that extends further down the mid shaft of the femur (short arrow) than is seen on the radiograph. Soft tissue involvement is also evident (arrowheads).

10.2 Arthritides

Arthritides are diseases of the joints. Joints can become pathological in a number of ways, so use an organised structured approach to differentiate the various diseases.

Key fact
- Arthritides fall into three broad disease categories on imaging: hypertrophic, erosive and infective.

Radiological findings

Radiographs of the small joints, typically of the hands, have characteristic features (**Table 10.3**). A common finding of most

Feature	Radiographic findings
Alignment	• Normal • Subluxation or deviation of digits
Bony changes	• Osteophytes • Subchondral sclerosis • Subchondral cysts (geodes) • Overhanging cortical edge • Periosteal new bone • Ankylosis of bone
Calcification	• Chondrocalcinosis • Tendinous calcification • Calcification of soft tissue (with or without a mass)
Mineralisation	• Normal • Juxta-articular or diffuse osteoporosis
Erosion	• Site of erosion • Aggressive (without reactive bone) or non-aggressive (with reactive bone)
Joint space	• Normal • Uniform or asymmetrical narrowing
Soft tissue swelling	• Symmetrical or asymmetrical around the joint • Lumpy bumpy • Diffuse (involving entire digit)

Table 10.3 Identifiable features in anteroposterior radiographs of the hands

arthritides is joint space narrowing. A differential diagnosis can be obtained by evaluating the pattern of joint space narrowing along with other characteristic features (**Figure 10.17**).

Radiography This remains the main modality for screening. A bilateral anteroposterior radiograph of the hands is taken for classic appearances. Radiographs of other joints, including those of the feet, hips, and knees, are done according to symptoms.

Ultrasound

This is used to determine if active synovitis is present. The results determine management.

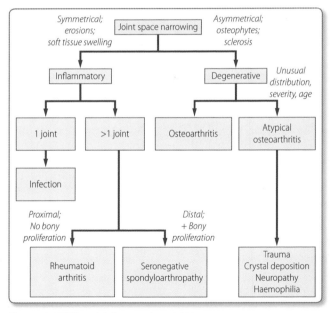

Figure 10.17 Differential diagnoses for arthritides.

Magnetic resonance imaging

This can be used for the early detection of arthropathic changes but is more often used as a research tool.

Key imaging findings

- Synovitis
- Erosions
- Focal bone marrow oedema

Treatment: Treatment depends on the type of arthritis and the site of arthropathy. Analgesics may be adequate for early disease. In long-term disease, joint replacement may be necessary. Inflammatory arthritides probably need anti-inflammatory treatment. Infectious arthritides need urgent management.

Hypertrophic arthritides

Degenerative primary and secondary osteoarthritis and Charcot's joint are hypertrophic arthritides.

Primary osteoarthritis

Primary osteoarthritis is intrinsic degeneration. The precise aetiology is unknown. The knees and hips (**Figure 10.18**) are affected more often than the elbows and shoulders. The disease affects 10 times as many women than men. The 1st metacarpophalangeal and distal phalangeal joints are typically affected (**Figure 10.19**).

Look for the triad of joint space narrowing, subchondral sclerosis and (marginal) osteophytes (Bouchard's nodes in the proximal interphalangeal joint or Heberden's nodes in the distal interphalangeal joint). A subchondral cyst (geode) is often also present.

Secondary osteoarthritis

Secondary osteoarthritis is destruction of the articular process by extrinsic causes. The disease occurs in patients at an age atypical for osteoarthritis. The location and appearance of the pathological changes are also atypical.

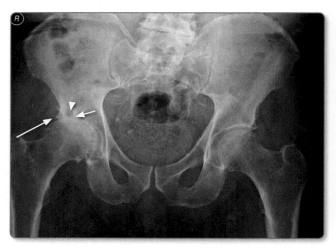

Figure 10.18 Anteroposterior radiograph of the pelvis, showing severe osteoarthritis on the right. Note the characteristic loss of joint space, subchondral sclerosis (short arrow) and osteophytes (long arrow). A subchondral cyst (geode) is present (arrowhead).

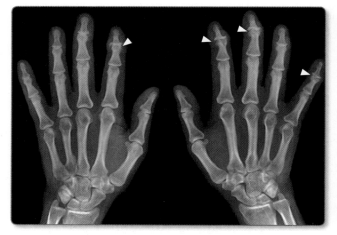

Figure 10.19 Bilateral anteroposterior radiograph of the hands, showing osteophytes, reduced joint spaces and subchondral sclerosis. These findings are typical of osteoarthritis at the distal interphalangeal joints (arrowheads). The metacarpophalangeal and proximal interphalangeal joints remain normal.

Trauma, infection, avascular necrosis, calcium pyrophosphate dihydrate deposition, rheumatoid arthritis, haemophilia, haemachromatosis, acromegaly and Wilson's disease can cause secondary osteoarthritis.

Charcot's joint

Charcot's joint is a neuropathic joint caused by abnormal sensation and proprioception leading to progressive joint destruction. Diabetes is the commonest cause.

Look for increased density (subchondral sclerosis), destruction, distension, dislocation, disorganisation and debris (intra-articular loose bodies) (**Figure 10.20**).

Erosive arthritides

Rheumatoid arthritis, gout, haemophilia, erosive osteoarthritis, seronegative connective tissue disease (scleroderma, systemic lupus erythematosus and sarcoidosis) and amyloidosis (rare) are all erosive arthritides.

Rheumatoid arthritis

Rheumatoid arthritis is bilateral and symmetrical. Pathological changes first appear at the metacarpophalangeal joint, proximal interphalangeal joint and ulnar styloid. The radiocarpal joint is commonly narrowed. Secondary degenerative

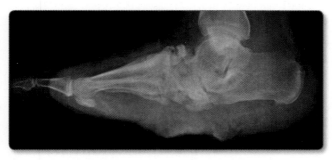

Figure 10.20 Lateral radiograph of the right foot, showing Charcot's joint resulting from destruction of the midfoot in a patient with diabetes. The classic 'rocker bottom deformity' is seen here.

arthropathy can occur, especially in the larger joints of the hips and knees.

Look for uniform joint space narrowing, marginal erosion, periarticular osteoporosis, fusiform soft tissue swelling and sub-luxations (**Figure 10.21**). Large joints typically have no erosion.

In secondary degenerative joint disease, there is marked nar-rowing, with an intact articular cortex and little sclerosis. Late-stage arthritis mutilans causes extensive destruction (**Figure 10.22**).

Gout

Gout is asymmetrical and monoarticular. It is more common in men. The metatarsophalangeal joint is usually affected first. Tophi rarely calcify. Olecranon bursitis is common.

Look for juxta-articular erosions; these are sharply margin-ated, with sclerotic rims. There is also an overhanging edge (so-called rat bite or punched-out lesions). Initially, no joint space narrowing is present, and there is little or no periarticular osteoporosis. Soft tissue swelling is visible (**Figure 10.23**)

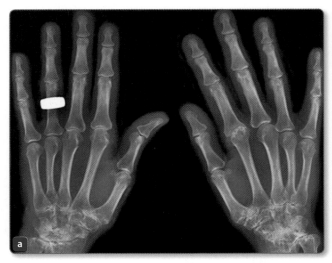

Figure 10.21a *For caption see opposite.*

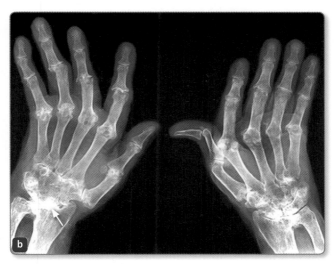

Figure 10.21b Bilateral anteroposterior radiographs of the hands, showing pathological changes caused by rheumatoid arthritis. (a) In the early stages, there is loss of joint space and erosion of the wrist joints (including the ulnar styloid) in both hands. Periarticular osteoporosis is also present. Similar changes are also visible in the metacarpophalangeal joint of the right index finger. (b) In the late stages, there is bilateral symmetrical involvement of the wrist and the metacarpophalangeal and proximal interphalangeal joints. Ankylosis of the carpal bones is visible on the left (arrow). Ulnar deviation is also present.

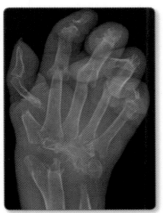

Figure 10.22 Anteroposterior radiograph of the right hand, showing arthritis mutilans. There is extensive destruction of the wrist and the metacarpophalangeal and proximal interphalangeal joints, with subluxations.

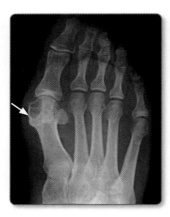

Figure 10.23 Anteroposterior radiograph of the right foot, showing juxta-articular erosion with sclerotic edges (arrow) and soft tissue swelling at the metatarsophalangeal joint of the hallux. These findings are consistent with gout.

Calcium pyrophosphate dihydrate deposition disease

Calcium pyrophosphate dihydrate deposition disease is idiopathic but is associated with hyperparathyroidism and haemochromatosis. The disease is symmetrical, and the knee is more commonly affected than the wrist (at the metacarpophalangeal joint). It has a sudden onset, with the joints becoming red and swollen.

Look for chondrocalcinosis, including in the triangular fibrocartilage complex and the symphysis, and large subchondral cysts, including in the patellofemoral joints (**Figure 10.24**).

Haemophilia

Haemophilia produces pathological changes in the large joints: haemorrhage, synovitis, pannus, hyperaemic response and bone resorption and remodelling (especially open epiphyses). Overgrowth of the epiphysis, resorption of secondary trabeculae (longitudinal striations), widening of the intercondylar notch, joint effusion and haemosiderin deposits may be present (**Figure 10.25**). The differential diagnosis is juvenile rheumatoid arthritis.

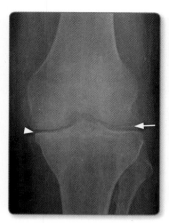

Figure 10.24 Anterior radiograph of the left knee, showing joint degeneration with reduced medial joint space (arrowhead) and chrondrocalcinosis (arrow) caused by calcium pyrophosphate dihydrate deposition.

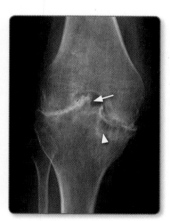

Figure 10.25 Anteroposterior radiograph of the right knee of a patient with haemophilia. The intercondylar notch is widened (arrow). Because of chronic joint destruction, degenerative changes with subchondral cysts are present (arrowhead).

Erosive osteoarthritis

Erosive osteoarthritis affects the interphalangeal and carpometacarpal joints of post-menopausal women. There is degenerative joint disease with marked inflammation and central erosions that resemble gull wings (**Figure 10.26**).

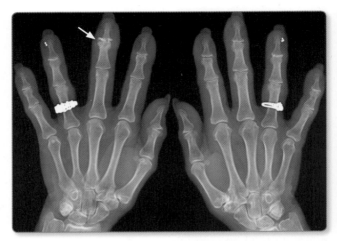

Figure 10.26 Bilateral anteroposterior radiograph of the hands, showing isolated central gull wing erosions of the distal interphalangeal joint of the left middle finger (arrow). This finding is consistent with erosive osteoarthritis.

Seronegative rheumatoid arthritis variants

These variants include negative rheumatoid factor and positive HLA-B27. Periarticular osteoporosis is usually absent, but periostitis (whiskering) is common (compared with rheumatoid arthritis, which invariably is accompanied by periarticular osteoporosis). Ankylosis is often present. Asymmetrical peripheral joint changes are visible.

Psoriatic arthritis

Psoriatic arthritis accompanies skin (especially nail) changes. The distal interphalangeal joints of the hands are affected more often than the joints of the feet. Peripheral lesions resemble mouse ears, and the disease can cause a pencil-in-cup deformity (**Figure 10.27**). Occasionally, resorption of the terminal phalanges (acro-osteolysis) and diffuse soft tissue swelling (so-called sausage fingers) occur. There is no periarticular osteoporosis.

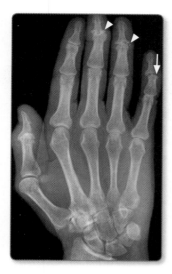

Figure 10.27 Anteroposterior radiograph of the right hand, showing psoriatic arthritis. Peripheral bare area erosions (arrowheads), called mouse ears, are visible in the distal interphalangeal joints of the middle and ring fingers. The distal interphalangeal joint of the little finger is starting to show the pencil-in-cup deformity (arrow).

Reiter's syndrome

Reiter's syndrome involve urethritis, arthritis (in 50% of cases) and conjunctivitis. The syndrome affects the feet more often than the hands, and it also affects the sacroiliac joint. Periostitis is present at sites of tendinous insertions. Periarticular osteoporosis can occur, similar to rheumatoid arthritis.

Ankylosing spondylitis

Most patients with ankylosing spondylitis are HLA-B27 positive. The disease involves bilateral sacroiliac arthritis and squaring of the vertebral bodies. Continuous syndesmophytes produce the characteristic bamboo spine appearance (**Figure 10.28**). Peripheral arthritis affects the large joints. MRI can detect the shiny corners of Romanus lesions in ankylosing spondylitis earlier than radiography can (**Figure 10.29**).

Enteropathic arthropathy

Enteropathic arthropathy can occur with ulcerative colitis or, less commonly, Crohn's disease. In the spine, the disease

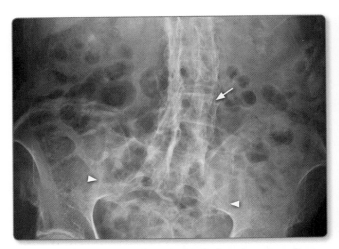

Figure 10.28 Anteroposterior radiograph of the lumbar spine and sacroiliac joint, showing flowing syndesmophytes (arrow) producing the bamboo spine appearance of ankylosing spondylitis. Bilateral sacroiliac joints have fused (arrowheads).

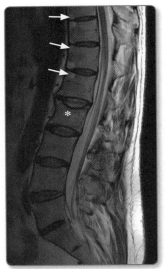

Figure 10.29 Sagittal T2-weighted magnetic resonance imaging of the spine, showing multiple areas of increased signal (arrows). These areas are the shiny corners of Romanus lesions, early erosive changes in ankylosing spondylitis. Note the grade 1 biconcave fracture of the L2 vertebra (*).

resembles ankylosing spondylitis. As in psoriatic arthritis, asymmetrical sacroiliitis is present, but in enteropathic arthopathy the peripheral joints have no erosions.

Infectious arthritides

Infectious arthritides are more common in adults than in children. In adults, the infection is more likely to arise from local trauma. Children get osteomyelitis. The infectious agent is typically *Staphylococcus aureus*. If the infection is tuberculosis, the disease has a protracted course. Tuberculous arthritis usually affects the spine in children; in adults, the knee is more commonly involved.

Infectious arthritides destroy the articular surface. They tend to affect one joint (unlike gout, which can affect multiple joints). Healing with ankylosis is common.

Radiographs are initially normal. Ultrasound may detect joint effusion (**Figure 10.30**). MRI can be used to look for adjacent bony involvement.

10.3 Paget's disease

Paget's disease of the bone was previously termed osteitis deformans. It is a common bone disorder in which abnormal bone resorption and remodelling result in osseous overgrowth and weakening.

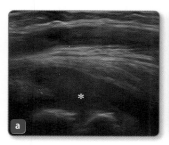 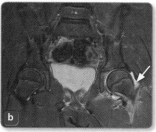

Figure 10.30 (a) Longitudinal ultrasound of the left hip of a 7-year-old child, showing increased joint effusion (*). The overlying tubular structure is the femoral artery. (b) Coronal STIR magnetic resonance imaging confirmed left hip joint effusion (arrow) without adjacent osteomyelitis. Joint aspiration confirmed septic arthritis.

Key facts

- The pelvis is most likely to be affected, followed by the femur, the skull, the tibia and the vertebrae. Most cases involve multiple bones.
- The cause of Paget's disease is unknown. The disorder is uncommon in patients younger than 40 years but affects 10% of people over the age of 80 years.
- Pathological fractures usually develop on the convex side of the bone and progress to become complete.
- Sarcomatous transformation occurs in less than 1% of patients. The process typically occurs over a long time, and it is commoner in patients with extensive polyostotic disease. The commonest sites for sarcomas to develop are the proximal femur, pelvis and shoulder.

Radiological findings

Paget's disease occurs in three phases:

1. The lytic (active) phase, in which excessive osteoclastic activity causes bone to be resorbed.
2. The mixed phase, in which bone is simultaneously resorbed and formed.
3. The blastic (late) phase, in which abnormal bone is formed.

The disease is usually diagnosed in the mixed phase. It gradually affects an entire bone but does not cross joint margins.

Radiography Long bones in the lytic phase of Pagets' disease initially have a subchondral lucency extending from the epiphysis to the diaphysis. The sharply defined lytic lesion has a flame or blade-of-grass shape (**Figure 10.31**). Cortical scalloping may be present. In a skull in the lytic phase of the disease, a well-defined circular lucency is visible in the inner calvarial table (osteolysis circumscripta).

Bones in the mixed phase show cortical thickening interspersed with lucencies and trabecular coarsening, usually along lines of stress such as the ilioischial and iliopectineal lines in the pelvis (**Figure 10.32**). The skull shows patchy, round sclerosis crossing sutures and resembling cotton wool (**Figure 10.33**). Affected vertebral bodies commonly have a picture frame appearance caused by thickening of the margins.

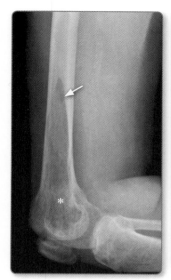

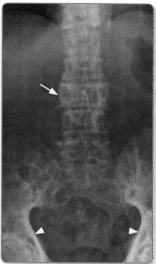

Figure 10.31 Lateral radiograph of the right femur, showing a lucency (*) extending from the epiphysis to the diaphysis. The lesion is sharply defined and shaped like a flame or blade of grass (arrow), which is characteristic of the lytic phase of Paget's disease.

Figure 10.32 Anteroposterior radiograph of the lumbar spine and sacroiliac joints, showing thickening of the ilioischial lines and iliopectineal lines (arrowheads). Paget's disease also involves the L3 vertebral body (arrow), which is enlarged.

In the blastic phase, extensive sclerosis with dense irregular trabeculae is visible in thickened and deformed bones. Long bones can become bowed. The bone tends to be larger overall (**Figure 10.34**). So-called ivory vertebra may develop because of the diffuse sclerosis and enlargement during this phase.

Computerised tomography Changes on CT are similar to those on radiography. Cortical destruction is a sign of sarcomatous changes.

Bone scan Hypervascularity increases activity on bone scan in all three phases of Paget's disease (**Figure 10.35**).

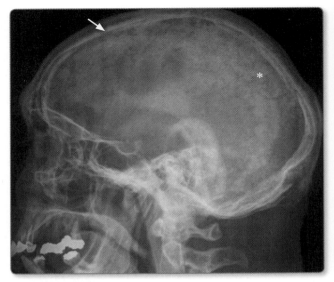

Figure 10.33 Lateral radiograph of the skull, showing mixed-phase Paget's disease. The cotton wool appearance (*) is caused by patchy, round sclerosis. The calvaria is thickened, more so in its inner table (arrow) than its outer table (in fibrous dysplasia, the outer table is more affected).

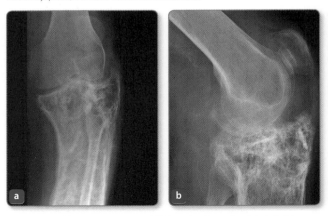

Figure 10.34 (a) Anteroposterior and (b) lateral radiographs of the left tibia, showing the mixed phase of Paget's disease. Irregular trabeculae are visible in thickened and deformed bones, which also show bowing.

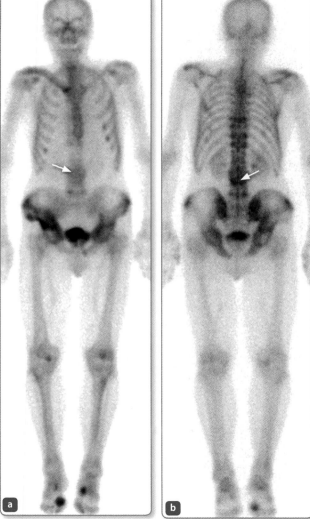

Figure 10.35 Isotope bone scans, (a) anterior and (b) posterior views showing increased uptake in the spine, including L3 vertebra (arrow) and pelvis. Degenerative uptake is visible in the feet.

However, in the late phase no excessive uptake may occur. Scintigraphic changes may be seen before Paget's disease is visible on radiography.

Magnetic resonance imaging   Bone in the lytic phase of Paget's disease shows heterogeneous hypointensity on T1-weighted MRI and hyperintensity on T2-weighted MRI. Small islands of residual marrow are often present. Bone in the mixed phase shows increased fat in the marrow (**Figure 10.36**). Bone in the blastic phase shows diffuse hypointensity on both T1-weighted and T2-weighted images. Cortical and trabecular thickening are more difficult to appreciate on MRI. Features of osteosarcoma may be present (see p.201).

Key imaging findings
- Lytic phase: look for flame-shaped or blade-of-grass long bones or osteolysis circumscripta of the skull, and intense uptake by the entire bone on bone scan.
- Mixed phase: the iliopectineal and ilioischial lines are thickened, the skull has a cotton wool appearance and the vertebrae may have a picture frame appearance.
- Blastic phase: bones are enlarged and deformed, and ivory vertebra may be visible.

Treatment
Treatment is symptomatic, with oral bisphosphonates to reduce pain. The surgical indication includes secondary neural compression or correction of the deformity. Malignant transformation into osteogenic sarcoma is rare (<1%) and has a poor prognosis.

10.4 Medullary bone infarcts

Medullary bone infarct involves loss of the trabecular pattern in the diametaphyseal medulla. Like avascular necrosis, this disorder is caused by ischaemia. However, medullary bony infarct has a different presentation from painful avascular necrosis involving physeal regions.

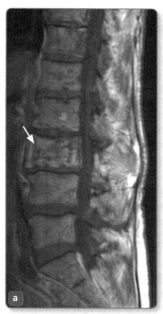
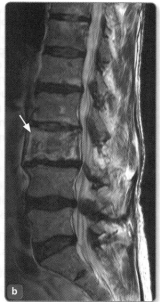
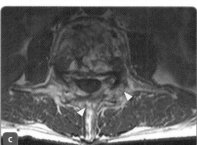

Figure 10.36 Sagittal (a) T1-weighted and (b) T2-weighted magnetic resonance imaging (MRI) of the lumbar spine, showing fatty (increased signal) and sclerotic (decreased signal) portions of the L3 vertebra (arrows). These findings are consistent with mixed-phase Paget's disease. (c) Axial T1-weighted MRI shows the disease extending to include the posterior elements (arrowhead). Same patient as Figure 10.35.

10.5 Osteomyelitis

Osteomyelitis is infection of the bone. Acute osteomyelitis occurs in abrupt clinical presentations. Chronic osteomyelitis occurs when there is a relapse or persistence of symptoms for > 6 weeks. Presentations vary. Acute osteomyelitis may present with the sudden onset of pyrexia and bone pain. In chronic osteomyelitis, the period between onset of symptoms and diagnosis may be longer.

Key facts

- The bone may be infected through haematogenous spread, contiguous spread or direct implantation (sometimes iatrogenic).
- The metaphysis of a long bone is the primary site of osteomyelitis in children. In adults, the most common sites are the pelvis, spine and long bones.
- In all age groups, the commonest causative organism is *S. aureus*, followed by *Streptococcus* organisms (usually the β-haemolytic *Streptococcus* species in children).

Radiological findings

Radiography Initial radiographs of affected areas show normal bones. However, soft tissue swelling with loss of fat planes is apparent within 3 days. Osseous involvement, that is, osteopaenia and medullary focal bony resorption, occurs 10 days after onset. Permeative bone destruction is a classic but non-specific sign of an aggressive lesion (**Figure 10.39**). Subacute osteomyelitis may result in a Brodie's abscess. The later chronic features are sequestra, involucrum and cloaca.

Computerised tomography Osseous changes are visible earlier on CT than on radiography. CT can also identify small foreign bodies, if present.

Bone scan Focal increased activity is found on all phases of a triple-phase bone scan in acute disease. Leucocyte scans can increase specificity (**Figure 10.40**).

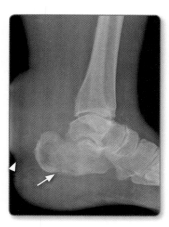

Figure 10.39 Lateral radiograph of the left ankle, showing the pathological fracture (arrow) and ill-defined permeative bony appearance of the calcaneum posteriorly. Ulceration (arrowhead) is present.

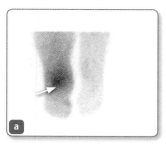 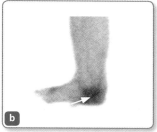

Figure 10.40 (a) Plantar and (b) longitudinal lateral leucocyte scans of the ankle, showing increased uptake in the posterior and inferior of the calcaneum (arrow) and surrounding soft tissue.

Magnetic resonance imaging Initially, non-specific marrow oedema is visible on MRI. This finding is followed by subacute soft tissue and osseous abscess, with other features of sequestra and sinus tracts. There is gadolinium enhancement of granulation tissue in the abscess wall and the sinus tract lining, as well as surrounding the non-enhancing sequestra (**Figure 10.41**). The sequestra remain low signal on all sequences.

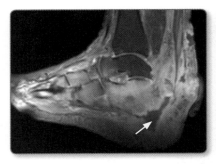

Figure 10.41 Sagittal post-contrast T1-weighted magnetic resonance imaging of the right ankle with fat suppression, showing increased signal in the calcaneum, with cortical bone loss and destruction posteriorly. There is an enhancing wall abscess (arrow) in adjacent soft tissue as well as pockets elsewhere.

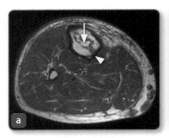
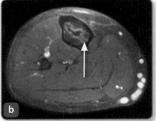

Figure 10.42 Axial magnetic resonance imaging with fat suppression. (a) T2-weighted image showing Brodie's abscess (arrow) in the medullary cavity of the right tibia. There is a communication via a cloaca through the periosteum (arrowhead). (b) T1-weighted image showing enhancing abscess walls and sinus tract (long arrow).

Key imaging findings

- Brodie's abscess is a well-defined metaphyseal lucency with a dense sclerotic rim (**Figure 10.42**).
- Sequestra are pieces of dense bone in an area of lucency caused by surrounding osteolysis.
- An involucrum is new bone formed by periosteal elevation and ossification (**Figures 10.43** and **10.44**).
- A cloaca is a sinus tract formed through periosteum or an involucrum.

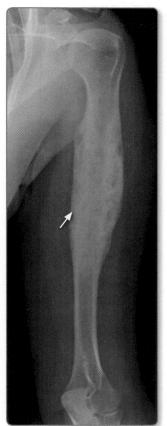

Figure 10.43 Anteroposterior radiograph of the left humerus, showing an involucrum (arrow), that is, new bone formed by periosteal elevation caused by chronic osteomyelitis.

- Look for the rim sign, a peripheral rim of low-signal fibrosis or sclerosis around affected marrow oedema in chronic osteomyelitis.

Treatment

Patients with acute osteomyelitis need intravenous antibiotics, usually for 4–6 weeks. Flucloxacillin and benzyl-penicillin usually cover the commonest organisms. Abscesses or chronic osteomyelitis usually need surgical debridement.

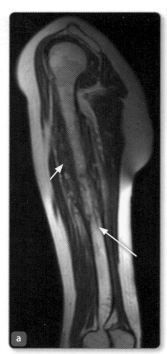

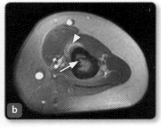

Figure 10.44 Magnetic resonance imaging (MRI) of the right humerus (same patient as in Figure 10.43). (a) Sagittal T2-weighted image showing an involucrum (short arrow) and a necrotic low-signal sequestrum (long arrow). (b) Axial T1-weighted MRI with fat suppression confirmed acute-on-chronic osteomyelitis (arrow) with adjacent soft tissue abscess formation (arrowhead).

10.6 Osteochondritis dissecans

Osteochondritis dissecans is the separation of a piece of articular cartilage and adjacent subchondral bone fragment from a joint surface. The name is a misnomer because there is no underlying inflammation of the bone or cartilage. The condition can affect any joint but particularly the elbows and knees.

Key facts

- Osteochondritis dissecans is more common in males than in females. It usually presents in adolescence but can also present in adults up to the age of 35 years.

- The cause is unknown but trauma may be the primary insult. Repeated microtrauma may cause the condition in some joints, such as the elbow.
- Ischaemia may be a secondary insult, with reduced blood flow leading to avascular necrosis of subchondral bone and articular cartilage.
- Bone and cartilage becomes fragmented. The loose bodies generated increase damage to the joint and cause further pain to the patient.

Radiological findings

Radiography Irregular joint changes with subchondral cystic features are visible on radiographs. Radiolucency can be present between the osteochondral defect and the underlying epiphysis (**Figure 10.45**). Detached fragments, if present, may appear as loose bodies, depending on the degree of ossification or calcification.

Computerised tomography The exact site and extent of the lesion can be detected using CT. CT is also useful for following the progression of osteochondritis dissecans. An irregular subchondral margin with cysts may be present. Smaller

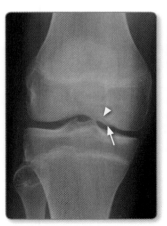

Figure 10.45 Anteroposterior radiograph of the right knee, showing the lucent rim (arrowhead) separating the osteochondral fragment (arrow) from the medial femoral condyle.

in the proximal humerus, distal radius, distal femur and tibial ends. Looser's zones are radiolucent short lines visible on the medial proximal femora, ribs and scapulae.

Key imaging findings

- Look for flaring, cupping and fraying of the metaphyses.
- A rachitic rosary is the expansion of the anterior rib ends.
- The legs bow on weight bearing.

Treatment

The aim is to treat the underlying cause with vitamin D replacement or phosphate supplements. Surgical correction is reserved for severe skeletal deformities.

Index

Note: Page numbers in **bold** or *italic* refer to tables or figures respectively.